50

FAT

AND

FRUSTRATED

What About **YOU?**

50

FAT

AND

FRUSTRATED
What About **YOU?**

GWENDOLYN C. JONES, Ph. D

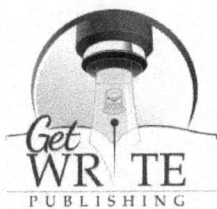

Get **WR** TE
PUBLISHING

50, Fat and Frustrated. What About You?
Copyright © 2018 by Gwendolyn C. Jones

Printed in the United States of America.

ISBN: 978-1-5323-9616-8

Editor:
Lisa Ann Johnson

Cover Design:
Kevin Vain, CoLab Creative Group

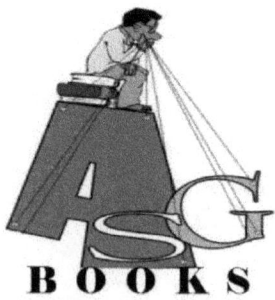

TABLE OF CONTENTS

ACKNOWLEDGEMENTS

To my wonderful parents; Henry E. Harris and Gloria M. Harris, and my grandmother, Mahala Gaskins Harris. And my other mother, Abna R. Hall. When the Lord takes me home for my rewards, I will remind him, it was because of each of you, I was able to complete the journey assigned to me. You started it and I will finish in the Lord. By the Grace of God!

To Mr. Elliott Smith, thank you for allowing God to use you.

To my aunts, Shirley Henderson and Ruth Dickerson, I love you for being my sister aunts.

To my sisters, Priscilla Williams and Selena Harris McQueen, and my late brother Roger Stratton, God kept us.

To John and Gloria Grimes, thanks for always being there for us.

To my children, John Love and Tameka Graham. The best is yet to come.

To God be all the Glory!

INTRODUCTION

Today many Christians struggle and are uncertain about their purpose and destiny in the earth. There is an unresolved desire to know more about their existence and what they should be doing as Christians. This lack of understanding of purpose can lead to an extended wilderness in life. This can also lead to depresssion, low self-esteem and comparing ourselves and our gifts and talents to others in the Body of Christ and or those in the world. It can also bring a spirit of jealousy for men and women alike who are competing with each other even though God made each of us uniquely different.

These comparisons are often seen in friendships, on the job, marriages, and in ministry. These are just a few problems and they are hindrances that can occur because of how we were raised, life experiences and things we are exposed to such as; trauma, afflictions, and our so-called "just life" experiences. These and many more incidents in our lives can delay our progression to our God-given destiny.

I defined wilderness as being busy doing everything or nothing besides what we are purposed to do for God. This wilderness is usually unintentional.

There were things in my life that kept me from fulfilling my God-given purpose because I was busy doing my own thing, not focused on my Christian walk or what I thought I should be doing because I couldn't locate my purpose. I knew I was supposed to do something, but it was so vague. I could not pinpoint or have a clear vision of my existence and my reason for being here. Even though I asked the Lord all the right questions, it seemed like such a long time to get the answers. I asked the who, what, when, where, and how about my existence.

Commit your works to the LORD
And your plans will be established.
Proverbs 16:3

God knew that in this world we must stay focused on our intended purpose and protect it with everything we have. He has already given us everything we need to accomplish his intended purpose for us.

Even though God allows trials and tribulations in our lives, He uses them to work together to help us to grow and mature in the faith. Therefore, all the life experiences must work together for our good and have a divine purpose that's attached to our destiny.

I am addressing just a few of the hindrances that can occur because of our family situations; how we were raised; things we are exposed to; trauma, afflictions, and our "just life" experiences. One thing for sure, we all are subject to encounters that can and will alter, change, or stop our God-given destiny.

However, if the truth is told, how do we accomplish our purpose if we are unsure of what it really is? We are here for an appointed time to do what we were sent here to accomplish according to God's will for each of us. We have been equipped with all that we need to accomplish

In this short period in life from birth until we leave this earth.

These things I have spoken unto you, that in me ye might have peace. In the world ye shall have tribulation: but be of good cheer; I have overcome the world.
John 16:33

In this book, I am sharing some of my "just life" experiences. I will show you some of the distractions or roadblocks that were placed before me from pre-birth. One of my main obstacles was in the area of my health; spirit, soul, and body; and how I was faced with many challenges that affected and delayed my purpose in the earth.

I will share how past health challenges exploded as I approached fifty. That's when the Lord helped me to take back control of my life when I found myself at 50, Fat, and Frustrated.

I will also share how those same experiences that almost destroyed me (and should have) were instead used to strengthen and propel me to success in Christ.

"And we know that all things work together for good to them that love God, to them who are called according to his purpose."
Romans 8:28

This autobiography is uniquely different from others. This book will help you get a clearer perception of your life experiences that are frequently unexplained. Experiences that may have occurred early in life, that might still have you in an unknown state of bondage and fear. These hindrances can often times prevent further progression in our personal, relational, ministry and business goals and objectives in life.

I will show you how to overcome the plan of destruction of your body or temple based on the word and power of God as the Holy Spirit reveals his health plan to change your life. It is called "divine health and healing." This will be done through Deliverance by the Holy Spirit as He illuminates the word of God in your past and present situations.

My prayer is that you will be able to identify any and all obstacles in your way, take control of them and move on to your destiny. We all need to get rid of anything that prevents us from our intended purpose so that we can live intentionally and reach that destiny.

When the Lord gave me this title and subject, I wondered why he wanted me to write about health in this way. He assured me that this topic is greatly needed in the Body of Christ.

There are too many people repeating patterns or staying in seats who should be running in this season.

The things that have happened to us have already been defeated and we need to get rid of them.

The Lord also wants me to bring out the goodness of God over the incidents so that we can walk in our victory successfully.

It is time to start tearing down those mindsets and take on the mind of Christ through His Word.

AN INCORRUPTIBLE INHERITANCE

We have an inheritance in Christ and now is the time to accept and receive the many treasures that God has in store for those who believe.

> **To an inheritance incorruptible, and undefiled, and that fadeth not away, reserved in heaven for you, Who are kept by the power of God through faith unto salvation ready to be revealed in the last time. Wherein ye greatly rejoice, though now for a season, if need be, ye are in heaviness through manifold temptations: That the trial of your faith, being much more precious than of gold that perisheth, though it be tried with fire, might be found unto praise and honour and glory at the appearing of Jesus Christ.**
> 1 Peter 1:4-7

God has already given us everything we need to accomplish His intended purpose for us. These treasures are kept and protected, and belong to His children. They are connected to our purpose.

As we come to the realization that Jesus is the only way and our answers are in the Lord and not in anyone or anything else, we obtain or received these gifts at the appointed time and season. We might have many and various temptations but, God uses them or turns them around to strengthen our faith walk. It's like going to school and taking an examination of what one learned all semester.

We stand before our Judge, Jesus, and He is looking for evidence that we passed the test with an A+. We not only got it but, by faith, we stand on it and move accordingly. No one can take that from us because we paid the price and it's fireproof.

On the other hand, if we don't pass the test, we have the opportunity to retake the class or wilderness experience until we do pass it. This can go on for many years. At least it did for me on several occasions. The goal is to have Father God say, "Well done" the first time.

The greatest thing about this test is that the answers are already available for us. We have all the answers. It's like waking up from sleep with mucus in your eyes; and it's hard to focus on what's before you. As you wipe your eyes and wash your face, you begin to regain focus.

Sometimes you may need a drop or two of Visine to help clear your vision. That's when our answers are revealed to us because we seek the face of God with clearer vision and understanding that He holds the answers. Everything we need related to our lives, existence, and purpose is right before us, but it takes focus.

We might even go through and stumble because things are not clear at first, but we have to keep going towards our Father God. This is called "working out our Salvation," there is no turning back.

My life experiences will help give you insight as to where brokenness comes from and what we need to get rid of the roadblocks in life. It will automatically set us up for healings to occur. We will also learn how to preserve, protect, and heal our temple God's way.

You will gain insight for your personal circumstances from situations I have experienced in my life; the trauma and the plan God already had in place to remove obstacles.

I will help you gain some basic knowledge of medical trends and terminology.

As you are released from many of these symptoms, you may notice improvement in some of the medical issues that are connected to spiritual and soulish symptoms also. Let go and let God do His thing.

You may also notice issues or similarities in your life that you will be able to pull the drawstring to connect the dots and bring the light of God on the scene.

Each chapter has a journaling section that will allow you to answer the thought-provoking questions you may have as the Holy Spirit speaks to you. Even though you might not know the answer, you do know that there is something that just won't let you move on in life. That thing that just keeps coming up in your spirit. It can be the feeling of low self-worth, rejection, lack of spiritual growth or lack of trust in God. It can also be related to living in fear, extreme phobias, anxiety, emotional eating or instability, traumatic events etc.

HIDDEN TREASURES

Therefore, God already wrote the answers to these treasures and they are in the Bible. It is our book of purpose. This book holds the things that are laid up for us that is safe, pure, and uniquely designed for each of us individually. Our books were written before we were birthed into the world. Everything about us and what and how we are to be and do was written down for us. Then we were formed and birthed.

Thine eyes did see my substance, yet being unperfect; and in thy book all my members were written, which in continuance were fashioned, when as yet there was none of them.
Psalm 139:16

Everything the Father has in store for us is written in a book and pre-ordained and pre-planned. We must come into agreement with what God wrote about us. This purposed plan is our holy calling, according to the will of God. He gives us the power and authority, gifting and talents, to do what we are designed to do. They are in heaven and just waiting for us to receive and walk in it. Praise God!

Who hath saved us, and called us with an holy calling, not according to our works, but according to his own purpose and grace, which was given us in Christ Jesus before the world began.
2 Timothy 1:9

However, if the truth is told, how do we accomplish our purpose if we are unsure of what it really is? We are here for an appointed time to do what we were sent here to accomplish according to God's will for each of us. We are equipped with everything we need to accomplish this short period in life from birth until we leave this earth.

**These things I have spoken unto you,
that in me ye might have peace. In the world ye
shall have tribulation: but be of good cheer;
I have overcome the world.**
John 6:33

The Holy Spirit is the one that will bring all things back to your remembrance. As we call on Holy Spirit, He will lead and guide you to all truth gently.

**If the Son therefore shall make you free,
ye shall be free indeed.**
John 8:32

Throughout this autobiography, there is an example of my own journey and experiences as a roadmap. There are five basic principles at the end of each chapter that will help you progress to the next level in your journey. They are:

Scarlet Thread Scripture - This indicates when the hand of God was there for you throughout your past and present experiences. Protecting and covering you when you didn't even realize it. Meditate on these scriptures.

Personal Reflection - You will think back to times, events, or feelings and emotions that present itself that causes a lack of peace or even fear. It can be noticed as a cycle event or episode that occurs every holiday, on your birthday or every month around the same time. It can even be that suicidal thought or plan just waiting for the right moment. It's that "something" that needs to GO!

Prayer: Ask the Holy Spirit to reveal what you need to know about that particular event or situation. Let Him lovingly expose the truth. Thank God for freedom and truth.

Personal Deliverance - Once exposed or taken out of darkness, you can have the Peace of God. You are released from that hold in your life.

Personal Renewal and Confession - Your God-intended purpose will be clearer as you live in your freedom. Be aware the problem might try to manifest itself again at a later date. Be persistent and go through the process until you fully tap into your VICTORY! Speak the Truth about who God says you are.

**Therefore if any man be in Christ,
he is a new creature: old things are passed away;
behold, all things become new.**
2 Corinthians 5:17

JOURNAL – WRITE YOUR INTRODUCTION

_____

_____

_____

_____

_____

_____

_____

_____

_____

_____

_____

_____

_____

_____

_____

_____

JOURNAL – WRITE YOUR INTRODUCTION

_____

_____

_____

_____

_____

_____

_____

_____

_____

_____

_____

_____

_____

_____

_____

_____

Chapter 1

THE BEGINNING

Many of my family members were born and raised in Washington, DC. (Native Washingtonians), including myself. A family of six in the1950s, we were far from middle class. I guess I can say we were a typical African American family living in Washington, District of Columbia; originating from the Foggy Bottom area in Northwest, DC.

When I was about seven years old, we relocated to subsidized housing in Southeast Washington and remained there for over 20 years.

We always had plenty of food to eat and pretty balanced meals, however, I grew up with a great dislike for vegetables. Regardless of the color of the vegetables, I really hated to eat them, especially, the green ones. Most of all, I knew that my body needed them. I also knew I would pay a great price for it later in life. My self-talk at that time was "you know you need that that healthy food, and "You're probably going to die young for not eating vegetables." I understood the connection between not eating healthy foods, early death, and sickness at a young age.

I will share some of the challenges I went through. I will share the journey I traveled from infancy to the present. I clearly see the brick and mortar and the cracks in the road now. The things that caused me to trip and fall for many years.

**"For I know the thoughts that I think toward you;
saith the LORD, thoughts of peace, and not of
evil, to give you an expected end."**
Jeremiah 29:11

The Lord opened my eyes to see and understand those pitfalls. My path is clearer because many of the road-blocks are removed.

EXPECTED END

Life was a real experience for me and I didn't know why or what it was all about or why things seemed so challenging. I just wanted love and happiness through-out my life. I asked the Lord often, "Why am I here in this horrible place on earth?" It was as if I'd known I came from somewhere else.

**And I set my mind to seek and explore by
wisdom concerning all that has been done under
heaven. It is a grievous task which God has given
to the sons of men to be afflicted with.**
Ecclesiastes 1:13

Finally, I got a hold of life and started to grow and function, however, I always wondered about the evil-ness upon the earth. I thank the Lord for showing me a clearer path or road that He prepared and intended for me to follow. This path was prepared and intended from heaven for me to accomplish here on earth.

I cried many tears for the Lord to show me the way. I knew what I had been through and I needed to know why I was placed in the earth. I knew I was supposed to be doing something. I just didn't know what it was. I needed answers. The answers I needed, only the Lord could answer. I needed to understand the "why" of my existence.

Each of us has a roadway or path that was prepared for us before the foundation of the world and is designed for us in Christ Jesus for God's Glory.

Then they cry unto the LORD in their trouble, and he saveth them out of their distresses. He sent his word, and healed them, and delivered them from their destructions.
Psalm 107:19-20

MEDICAL STUMBLING BLOCKS

I experienced many medical issues throughout my life. Some were physical and other symptoms are emotional or spiritual. Some of my problems came from just not eating the right foods to fuel my body and not properly caring for my body. However, I must note that as an infant born with an inner deficit, it was a blind battle I was coming up against. The knowledge of today was not available over 60 years ago but the same problems were.

The Word of God says, "We are born in sin and shaped in iniquity." I will share some of the challenges I went through as a child and my personal journey from my beginning until my adult life. I will also share how I experienced many illnesses and how they presented itself in my spirit, soul, and body.

**For I was born a sinner—yes,
from the moment my mother conceived me.**
Psalm 51:5

I clearly see the bricks laid and the cracks in the road that caused me to stumble early in life. The things that caused me to trip and fall for many years are the very incidents that the Lord opened my eyes to see and understand as pitfalls and how I am an overcomer of them all because I already have the victory in Jesus Christ.

As I search for many answers, Father God began to reveal to me answers and solutions. My path is clearer because many of the old roadblocks are removed and a new foundation laid. This new foundation is in Christ Jesus who is the Deliverer of my spirit, body, and soul. Praise God!

**See, I have this day set thee over the nations and
over the kingdoms, to root out, and to pull down,
and to destroy, and to throw down,
to build, and to plant.**
Jeremiah 1:10

In the above scripture, the Lord asked Jeremiah what did he see before him as his purpose and mission. I see this process of life afflictions before our born-again experience as the work of the enemy inflicting us in our infancy in an attempt to stop the ministry and work and ministry of Jesus in the earth.

For Christ also hath once suffered for sins, the just for the unjust, that he might bring us to God, being put to death in the flesh, but quickened by the Spirit.
1 Peter 3:18

I love how this scripture shows how Christ suffered for the sins of the unjust too, that was me and you before our salvation experience. It also tells us how one can get through the stumbling blocks the enemy bring our way and that we won't continue to trip up when trying to live a faith-filled life after salvation. This verse says He puts them to death in the flesh, so our spirit man can come alive in Christ, removing the hindrances. Praise God!

The Lord is saying that we have the authority over the kingdom of darkness and have the ability to root out this affliction, to pull down the strongholds, and to destroy the power of darkness from operating in our lives. Then we can begin to build and plan the seed of faith inside of us for health and fulfillment in Christ Jesus for the Glory of God.

I thank the Lord for showing me my new life in Christ which is the clear path or road that He prepared for me to follow. This path was prepared and intended from heaven for me to accomplish on earth during my period of time here called "Life." Each of us has a roadway or path that was prepared by God for His Glory to be manifested in and through us. This pathway is our purpose, designed before the foundation of the world and is embedded in us to be discovered as we walk closer to the Lord.

Then shall the King say unto them on his right hand, Come, ye blessed of my Father, inherit the kingdom prepared for you from the foundation of the world.
Matthew 25:34

INTERCEPTORS

There are many things that can interfere with the plan and purpose for your life as God intended. My primary focus in this book is in the area of our health; spirit, soul, and body.

We have many obstacles when it comes to our physical temple that I think is often overlooked. It is not acknowledged as a problem because I believe we don't see it as a real hindrance to our mission in life.

When I was challenged with the inability to move, think clearly, feel energetic, aches and pains, inferiority complex and just an overall bad feeling myself, I felt threatened. I really didn't understand what was happening to me.

Therefore, I believe one's health can be a great interceptor as almost anything else. It's time to pay more attention to this enemy within, that has crept into the body of Christ that can alter your destiny.

We also have a responsibility to take care of our temple. That is our whole man, spirit, soul, and body. Therefore, to neglect ourselves is a definite interceptor.

I really believe I was my own biggest problem in my youth and early adult life. My poor dietary habits made matters worse.

Another hindrance was my soul or mind, will, intellect, and emotions. This can come in the form of listening to words that others say about us that are opposite of the word of God. We are to resist negative words that come within our hearing.

Lastly, another hindrance I had was in the realm of the spirit. This was seen in low self-esteem, inferiority complex, abandonment, fear, and anxiety.

I want to discuss first, that we definitely have an enemy. The enemy's job is to present crossroads and stumbling blocks before us. He will attempt to intervene and bring confusion that can change, delay, or even kill our purpose in God.

The thief cometh not, but for to steal, and to kill, and to destroy: I am come that they might have life and that they might have it more abundantly.
John 10:10

On the other hand, this world system may have processes in place that can prevent us from tapping into our full potential, especially if we are walking more by sight instead of faith. All of these interventions can make it difficult for us to understand and walk in purpose.

When I connected the journey from my beginning, I was able to see and understand myself like never before. I also made incredible, immediate changes in my thoughts and behavior, understand and love myself and others. I had a clearer vision of my God-intended purpose and how the enemy had other plans for my life.

God opened my eyes to see how the enemy meant to destroy me. He kept me and delivered me. Praise God!

Our God Turns Around the Negative to Positive

We are blind until God opens our spiritual eyes. It is now time for an awakening of our spirit, soul and body connection and interconnection. There are many traumatic experiences that occur as we walk this journey called "Life." These distractions may cause us to go off course from our God-given purpose and destiny, but we have a deep well to draw from and that well is Christ Jesus.

In the next chapter, I will show you some examples of my life experiences of trauma and what was certainly meant to take me out. But God!

The enemy comes to kill, still, and destroy us in our infancy. Remember they tried to kill the Baby Jesus.

**"For Herod will seek the young Child
to destroy Him."**
Matthew 2:13b

Many of us experienced things as an infant and early childhood years in an attempt to destroy us. These attacks can come in the form of all types of abuse; rape, physical, emotional, or spiritual. Other forms are stress and anxiety, mental deficits, and many other disguises. We can no longer let issues set us down on our journey or stop us in our tracks. We are over-comers. Like Jesus, I am determined not to die before my time.

"I shall not die, but live,
and declare the works of the LORD."
Psalm 118:17

ROADMAP TO VICTORY!

<u>Scarlet Thread Scripture</u> – What experience or scripture reference is the Holy Spirit giving you concerning your early life issues or situations? Meditate on that scripture.

_____

<u>Personal Reflection</u> - Think back to a time that you first noticed an unusual feeling, behavior, or thought; a lack of peace or, even fear, early in life. What is the Holy Spirit revealing to you?

_____

_____

<u>Prayer</u> - Ask the Holy Spirit to reveal what you need to know. Let Him lovingly expose the truth.

_____

_____

_____

<u>Personal Deliverance</u> - Once exposed or taken out of darkness, the Lord will remove its power. You will have Peace! Did you receive your peace? _____

<u>Personal Renewal and Confession</u> - Now you can move on from that crack in the road. This crossroad can and is removed.

JOURNAL – WRITE YOUR BEGINNING

_____

_____

_____

_____

_____

_____

_____

_____

_____

_____

_____

_____

_____

JOURNAL - WRITE YOUR BEGINNING

_____

_____

_____

_____

_____

_____

_____

_____

_____

_____

_____

_____

_____

_____

_____

_____

Chapter 2

MY PRE-BIRTH EXPERIENCE

As an infant, my beloved mother, Gloria Mildred Harris, was stricken with Tuberculosis and in the 1940's and she was admitted to the hospital for treatment. This was sometime between the birth of my brother, Gary, and sister, Priscilla. My family lived in the Georgetown area of Washington, DC, at that time.

This was a very traumatic period for my family. I recently discovered this information from my Aunt Ruth, that my mother was initially diagnosed and treated for Tuberculosis or TB before I was born. I never knew that all these years. I was too young to ask any questions before my mother passed away and just didn't know what to ask my father who passed away suddenly.

> Tuberculosis was a problem everywhere in the 1930s, but the disease hit few places as hard as it hit Washington, D.C. While it might have been true that many parts of Washington was not as congested as other cities, a large proportion of the population – primarily poor blacks – lived in overflowing alley settlements.
>
> DC's TB Problem 2/10/2015 in DC, Maryland by Mark Jones

My mother relapsed when I was about six months old and was hospitalized again. Though I don't remember this time in my life, I do know the effects I experienced emotionally, physically, and spiritually. These experiences appeared to have exploded when I was leading up to my 50th birthday. That's how I got the title of my book, *50, Fat and Frustrated.*

I want to help you discover some answers for your own situations. Hopefully, you will be able to see some connections from your past that might have an influence on your life today.

THE TRAUMA

My mother was severely ill for a while before I was born as I mentioned. She was admitted into Glenn Dale Sanatorium in Prince Georges County, Maryland. The treatment at that time was isolation and many new TB-fighting antibiotics were developed during that period.

One of her treatments was the iron lung machine. "This was an equalizing pressure chamber which enables the patient to stop breathing!" This treatment allowed the lungs to rest.

> *Washington Post* expose explained: **"Tuberculosis is the curse of the alleys. There is not enough light and there is not enough air... Disease starts in the alleys and it spreads...**
>
> Boundary Stones WETA'S Local History Blog

I am a product of her cervical-vaginal environment or the tiny life system within her womb that kept me nourished and alive. Within my mother's spirit, soul and body were stress, fear, anxiety, feelings of isolation and depression which is usually connected to chronic illness and a lowered immune system.

CONCEPTION

The tuberculosis went into remission and my mother came home from the hospital. It didn't take too long before I was conceived. Now let's take a closer look at what happens in the womb when it comes to genetics transfer from mother to infant.

Treatments for tuberculosis during that time were intense with surgery, antibiotics, and isolation as mentioned. I am quite sure all of these treatments were necessary, however, what effect did this stress have on my mother and what was genetically passed on to me at conception? Is it impossible to give something you don't have (ex. good health)? Can a mother pass on what she is experiencing in her own health to her infant inside of her?

Needless to say, my mom's immune system wasn't as strong as it could have been because of her illness and the therapeutic treatments for TB. Can you imagine what was passed on to me?

> **Genetics is a branch of biology; the science of heredity, dealing with resemblances and differences of related organisms resulting from the interaction of their genes and the internal environment.**
>
> Dictionary.com

What was the condition of my immune system as a result of my mother's illness? Would this affect my life after birth? Did I have any signs or symptoms that would indicate I had a few problems going on inside of me as an infant? Remember, this started before conception.

I also need to discuss the surroundings that I lived in while I was forming inside of her. This was my environmental life in the womb. This living condition in the womb helped establish my genetic makeup because I ate, breathed, moved, and lived in her womb for nine months. Science says that we are made up from our parent's genetics and environment. This discovery in science identifies how environment plays a very important part in our overall makeup. This is called epigenetics.

> **Epigenetics (Summary): Research into epigenetics has shown that environmental factors affect characteristics of organisms. These changes are sometimes passed on to the offspring.**
>
> DNA Isn't Everything April 13, 2009 ETH Zurich

By the way, my sister Priscilla is just a year and a half older than me. I was informed that my mother was initially ill before my sister and I were born. However, the disease returned after I was a few months old.

Mom was admitted to Glenn Dale, this time for several years. She was put on what was called an Iron Lung breathing machine to rest her lungs so they could heal. This was also extremely traumatic for her.

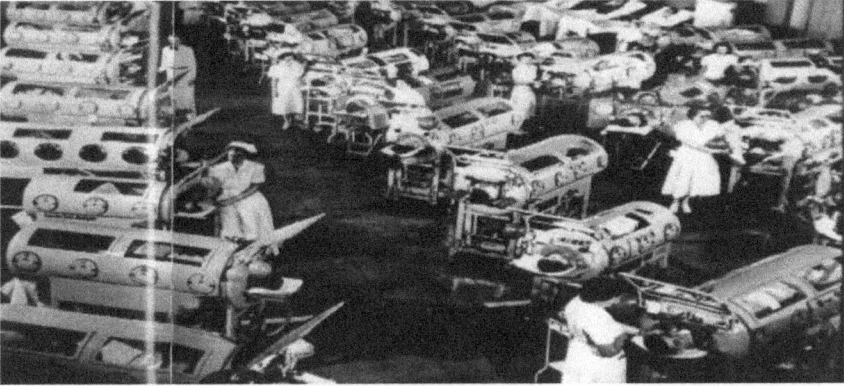

In 1959, there were 1,200 people using tank respirators in the United States; in 2004, there were 39.

http://ariwatch.com/VS/TheIronLung/RespirationWithoutBreathing.html

Glenn Dale was not just for adults. Initially, it was a facility just for children. Many children contracted the disease—usually from the parents, caretakers or environment. I was my mother's baby at that time and was probably the closest person that had direct contact with her over an extended period of time before she was re-diagnosed with TB the second time. I never contracted TB from my mother, neither did anyone else in my family. Praise God for his covering and protection!

FAMILY SECRETS

But when it pleased God, who separated me from my mother's womb, and called me by his grace.
Galatians 1:5

Many of us have stories of our childhood and some of them may be family secrets and hidden stories that never been told. When I was a child, children were not supposed to ask questions. Because of that culture in many African-American families, there are many things that are still family secrets that are unknown or unspoken.

It is important to know what medical diagnoses, psychological issues, suicides or murders, sexual abnormalities, emotional instability, inability to progress in life, physical tendencies, abusive events and most of all, generational signs. We must look at anything that might have an effect on your life.

Many of these things are hidden. One way to get answers is to start asking questions of family, friends, and associates. That is just exactly what I did and have been doing for many years now.

As I show you how I was able to trace just a few of my issues, many of them were revealed to me by the Lord as I began to study medical and scientific studies that are now being done and how they are related to my overall state of health today.

CONCLUSION

In this chapter, we discussed pre-birth and searched for minor things that could be affecting our adulthood in ways that could affect our path in life. It could be from hereditary or environment. These behaviors or attitudes could come from hidden things in our memory, our genetics epigenetics (environment), and are visible from the inside out. It's time for discovery and release by the Power of God!

In the next chapter, God is showing us a more excellent way. We will see how He has given us everything we need for survival. That He is the maker of the genes and controls the outcome as we lean on him. Praise God!

ROADMAP TO VICTORY!

<u>Scarlet Thread Scripture</u> – What scripture is the Holy Spirit giving you concerning your pre-birth experience? Ask about family secrets, occurrences, or habits. Meditate on the Scripture.

<u>Personal Reflection</u> – Think about occurrences that cause a lack of peace or even fear. Ask family and close friends for answers. Talk about those family secrets. No one is shamed but the devil.

<u>Prayer</u> – Thank you, Father God that you know all things. I ask for wisdom to know my genetic (parents) and epigenetic (environment) makeup, reveal family secrets, fears, unexplained emotions, etc.

<u>Personal Deliverance</u> - Allow the Holy Spirit to expose the truth. Once exposed or taken out of darkness, the Lord will remove its power. You will have Peace!

JOURNAL - WRITE YOUR PRE-BIRTH STORY

_____

_____

_____

_____

_____

_____

_____

_____

_____

_____

_____

_____

_____

JOURNAL – WRITE YOUR PRE-BIRTH STORY

_____

_____

_____

_____

_____

_____

_____

_____

_____

_____

_____

_____

_____

_____

Chapter 3

GOD AS FATHER / THE GENETIC DESIGN

Let's explore the genetic design of God as our Father. We know we have an earthly father, but we need to know that we have a spiritual father as well.

God as Father is important because we are who we are because of Him. We are made in His likeness. We get our genetic makeup from our parents, but we get our completeness of who we are as a spiritual being from Daddy God. Therefore, we are spirit first. We were handpicked and selected by God.

Father God formed me not only as a physical but also spiritual being. I was known of by the Father and had a relationship with Him before I was born. I was formed, and shaped for perfection.

Before I formed you in the womb I knew you.
Jeremiah 1:5

FORMED - yâtsar, yaw-tsar'; probably identical with H3334 (through the squeezing into shape); (compare H3331); to mould into a form; especially as a potter; figuratively, to determine (i.e. form a resolution):—× earthen, fashion, form, frame, make(-r), otter, purpose .The KJV translates Strong's H3335 in the following manner: form (26x), potter (17x), fashion (5x), maker (4x), frame (3x), make (3x), former (2x), earthen (1x), purposed (1x).

Strong's Concordance

Father God knew me and I had relationship with Him before I was born. I was then formed, shaped, and given a purpose. We all are frame and uniquely different. Genetics are not only derived from humans (our parents), but also divinely from God. This work was done from the creation of the world for all men and incorporated into our makeup at conception. We are not an afterthought but, we are preordained, predetermined, planned and purposed for his glory!

Word Origin: Root to Know
familiar friend (1), find (5), found (1), gain (1), had knowledge (1), had relations (6), had...relations (1), has (1), has regard (1), has...knowledge (1), have (4), have relations (3), have...knowledge

Strong's Concordance, 3045. yada

UNUSUAL BIRTH

Why was my birth unusual as well as yours? There is no such thing as routine. The word of God says we are all different. We are all the work of His hand and He made us before bringing us from eternity to time.

What is the price of two sparrows—one copper coin? But not a single sparrow can fall to the ground without your Father knowing it. And the very hairs on your head are all numbered. So don't be afraid; you are more valuable to God than a whole flock of sparrows.
Matthew 10:29-31

We are specially designed for the Master. He watch-es over us and keeps a count of every hair on our head and more. Praise God!

Well, my mother was severely ill for a while before I was born. Treated during this season then came back home. She was under a lot of stress in the hospital.

Mother went into remission, came home from the hospital and I was conceived. I was impacted both before and after my birth into the earth. My birth was a traumatic birth. Before I was born, I experienced severe stress. I was bathed in an atmosphere that was a challenge to survive.

After birth, life got even more stressful. I was born into an atmosphere that was even more of a challenge. I am sure before my mother knew the TB was back, she kept me very close to her as her newborn baby. I was the closest person to her. Wrapped in stress, tension, fear, and the chance of contracting TB myself. This was an "unusual birth."

According to as he hath chosen us in him before the foundation of the world, that we should be holy and without blame before him in love.
Ephesians 1:4

God knew me and you before we were ever made in the womb. He assigned my parents. He understood and knew me intimately and what my pre-life in the world would be like. And yet, He still placed me in the loving womb of my mother. Many would think, *why would God do that if she was ill?* Why in an environment that could possibly harm an embryo? Then God revealed to me the answer, the "Scarlet Thread." The blood of Jesus protected me as a fetus. God made me and formed me. As the Potter taking his loving hands and forming the clay and designing me for destiny. This was an indication of "This one is first." I can just hear the Lord saying, "This one will live for me." "This one is mine." Hallelujah!

God is looking for those that are the "first." Those that will live for Him and in Him. The Lord said to me, *"Look not at the thing that is around you. Stay focused on me and I will deliver you from all the works of the adversary."*

Father God loves us so much that He went to our ending and established our beginning. He is so precise that He took care of everything we needed in advance. He had it set up and determined and accomplished before the foundation of the world.

When I was really trying to figure this thing out concerning my existence, the Lord said to me, *I have called you before the foundation of the world."* Now, that really encouraged me and motivated me. I realized there are many like me that were placed in circumstances early in life that we had no control over.

Most times we may not even realize the things we went through, but we see symptoms manifesting in our spirit, soul, body, and especially emotional state in the forms of fear, anxiety, emotional eating, etc. We may appear as a mess to others, but did God make a mess?

So God created man in his own image, in the image of God created he him; male and female created he them.
Genesis 1:27

And God saw every thing that he had made, and, behold, it was very good.
Genesis 1:31a

We can point out or identify as well as others our personality quirks, fears, and anxieties, up and down emotions, eating disorders, addictions, clingy relationships, low self-esteem, unknown jealousy, and so on. Most of the time we just blame these manifestations on "it runs in my family." Well, you could be absolutely right.

I was fortunate to have my aunts and family friends tell me my story. You too can start asking questions about those things you hold on to for whatever reason. They could very well be the hindrances to your next level of your purpose. It is time to be set free!

What does it really mean before the foundation of the world?

Who hath saved us, and called us with an holy calling, not according to our works, but according to his own purpose and grace, which was given us in Christ Jesus before the world began.
2 Timothy 1:9

Jesus was slain before creation as it is written in the word of God. We are aware that we came from somewhere and Jesus is our example-setter or the first fruit.

We are also aware that our book of life was written with our purpose in it before we came to Earth. If God is a spirit and Jesus was a spirit without a body before He came to Earth, what does the scripture say about us? Are we a spirit man first?

Thine eyes did see my substance, yet being unperfect; and in thy book all my members were written, which in continuance were fashioned, when as yet there was none of them.
Psalm 139:16

Your eyes looked upon my embryo, and everything was recorded in your book. The days scheduled for my formation were inscribed, even though not one of them had come yet.
Psalm 139:16 – ISV

Praise God, He made us in such a miraculous way that man is still trying to figure it out. We were yet unformed substance and God wrote in His book of our life and purpose. Our birth date, to the second, was scheduled and documented.

This reality really encouraged me to know, in spite of issues in my life, I am not a mistake. I was planned and purposed in advanced by the Master. God knew what I would look like, the very hairs on my head, my fingerprints etc. What a wonderful, detailed Father. He made me just like Him. Hallelujah!

Your eyes saw my unformed substance, and in Your book, all the days [of my life] were written before ever they took shape, when as yet there was none of them.
Psalm 139:16 - AMPC

The best part is all this was done before we were assembled and our days on Earth were written. We have a purpose and that purpose is limited by time to discover and do it. Let's get started. Hallelujah!

GOD KNOWS ABOUT OUR PAIN

The turmoil we experience in life is not unknown to God. As we work through the trials and tribulations, we gain knowledge and trust for our Father every step of the way. This is how we grow our faith and are able to stand on the Word.

In the verse below, we see how God revealed to the wisest man to ever live, King Solomon, in his later years the pain and suffering of man and that we are to work it out in Christ.

I have seen the travail, which God hath given to the sons of men to be exercised in it.
Ecclesiastes 3:10

God gave him the wisdom to see the state of those who are trapped in this world system. Every man has God's genetic design within. That means we have the ability to know Him. He is not hiding from us, we just need to seek Him His way.

IT IS WRITTEN

We also know and believe that we are a tri-fold being. We are a spirit that has a soul and we live in a body suit. The bodysuit gives us permission to function in the earth. We need to start paying more attention to this bodysuit because it keeps us here on Earth. Without it, the bodysuit expires, and we go back to eternity. All spirits need one. Our purpose is for us to do the work of the Lord God in the earth as long as we can. We don't want to die a premature death.

When I was born in the earth, I came as an infant prepared to conquer the world. I came with attitude! I came with a purpose and a destined end. It was all genetically inside of my every gene. I was coded this way and I just didn't know it. My purpose had to be discovered and my God had to reveal it from the inside out. I was on a journey and so are you.

GOD'S GENETIC BLUEPRINT

To my discovery, as I was looking back at my path in life, I realized there were many crossroads and paths that were placed before me. Many were very painful and life alternating. I noticed many changes in who I became as I pioneered life, or you can say "discovered life." Having to adjust and change according to environmental conditions due to the existence of sin in the world. I came to the conclusion that life is an experience that just happens as we continue to live. In other words, *we don't know life but experience it.*

The good and bad, the happy and the sad, we live it. As a result of our exposures and experiences, we become who we are and discover our destiny. Our ultimate goal is to connect to God. This life journey is all about a journey to discover the true and living God and the purpose He places in us to work out on the earth for His Glory! The end result should be to know the Lord thy God and love Him with all your heart.

The greatest thing we will ever learn in life is to know we are lost without God. You see, Father God has placed in all of us His DNA. When He placed His breath of life in us and we became a living soul, He placed a desire within to know Him. This knowing is intimacy. We are made for Him. To be loved and communed with Father God and Him alone. What is man? Why do You love us so much, Lord?

HIDDEN COUNSEL

When God placed the world or eternity in our heart and gave us a large vision that included everything about Himself that could possibly be discovered. Then God put restrictions on the understanding until He decided the time for revealing in our individual lives. Therefore, we are counseled one-on-one and it is hidden within each of us. Just like our purpose is personal and only the Father can reveal it from the inside out, so is His purpose. As we work out our own salvation, we will develop our intimate relationship one-on-one with God! He is the one that is leading and directing us every step of the way to His purpose and Glory.

**He hath made every thing beautiful in his time:
also he hath set the world in their heart, so that
no man can find out the work that God maketh
from the beginning to the end.**
Ecclesiastes 3:11

These are the hidden works that God has done from the beginning to the end. It has all been laid out for us to work out our purposes, however, we cannot fully comprehend it all. It is too large, it is endless. In fact, it is hidden in eternity and we are eternal beings. We must seek God to find it.

This genetic formula is in man not animals or trees, but mankind that is made after the image of God. We are His children. He put the world in our heart, this is our genetic makeup of God to mankind.

Therefore, when we are going through the challenges in life, this is the epigenetic or environmental influences.

God is with us as we are working out our salvation since there is a time for every purpose under the sun. According to this verse, God is saying that both the timing and purpose is beautiful. This is an epigenetic state. We might call it terrible when we are going through tough times; however, the truth of this verse says that's not so.

As we grow in the Lord, we become more intimate with the Father, and He reveals who He is and who we are. He also reveals His work and purpose, and ours from the beginning to the end. Praise God!

All mankind got their genes from the one who made the genes. In Ecclesiastes, we see the genetic code 20:3:11. This code is expressed in the work of God in the earth from the beginning to the end.

We see how God made everything beautiful in its season and time. However, for man, He placed the world, or some translations say, "eternity in our heart." It is difficult for us to be fully able to grasp just how magnificent God really is or the completeness of His work.

This glory is for us to know that God is in control. However, we do have a glimpse of His wondrous glory demonstrated in His creation as we look around us. This glory is to us and for us. We can even see God's glory in ourselves and in one another.

Your hands made me and fashioned me; Give me understanding, that I may learn Your commandments.
Psalm 119:73

We are eternal beings just like our Father. God gave us the understanding, that we may learn and obey His laws.

In the numbering system of the Bible, we have the genetic code 20:3:11. This code allows us to see God with our spiritual eyes and perceive with our spiritual mind and believe Him in our heart. We can actually see His glorious handiwork in the world and know that God is real. We know just how great He is and how He cares for us out of His attributes, for God is Love.

Genetic Code 20:3:11

20 = 10X2 completion

3 = completion

11 is significant for disorder, chaos and judgment

Within this genetic code, 20:3:11, we can actually see just how God made everything beautiful in His time so hath set the world or eternity in the heart of man.

That's our very being or essence of who God is and who we are. We are not able to fully comprehend all the work God has done from eternity to destiny but, He reveals it in seasons, so we will know Him as we grow from glory to glory. I call this the genetic code 20:3:11 that is within the genetic makeup of mankind.

I would like to further explain the decoding this gene for a moment. The 20 is 10X2. This represents the completion of a waiting person or someone that is searching and is focused on their intimate relationship with the Father. This is our growth process as we mature in faith and wait on the Lord. The number three is also completion. It is how God reveals to us, more and more of the fullness of His existence and His work as we seek Him.

However, the number 11 means disorder, chaos, and judgment. This represents what we experience as we are in this world. The things we go through until we come in alignment with God. We must come in order with His will for our life.

When we walk in disobedience or before our Christ state, we are influenced greatly by our environment or epigenetics. We walk in lawlessness or become law-breakers, that is disobedience to the Word of God. We allow this world system to rule us instead of the Holy Spirit to lead and guide. However, God has designed us for His glory! He gave all mankind his genetic make-up.

---

11 Coming after 10 (which represents law and responsibility), the number eleven represents the opposite - the irresponsibility of breaking the Law, which brings disorder and judgment.

http://www.biblestudy.org/bibleref/meaning-of-numbers-in-bible/11.html

---

Let's focus on the One that makes the genes. What happens if we stay in a state of lawlessness? If we continue to be satisfied with the milk of the Word? If we do not grow in Christ? If we continue to live in our self-righteous state instead of dying to self?

What if we decide to hold on to those weights and don't give up the unforgiveness, anger, fear, frustration, etc. when prompted by the Holy Spirit?

There are the things that can move in the place of Jesus on the throne of our hearts that can bring judgment, chaos, and more disorder in life.

To conclude, the most powerful gene is from God. He placed His gene inside of us when He made us like Himself and gave us His life. We didn't make ourselves, we have a Creator that is larger than mere man.

Yes, we go through things in life but it is written in our hearts who we really are and our purpose in the earth. Therefore, we are to die to self, seek God and allow His hidden counsel as we go from glory to glory with our Maker.

In the next chapter, we will go back into the hidden areas of our life and look at some of the deeper symptoms and get rid of them because they are designed to stop us in our tracks.

ROADMAP TO VICTORY!

Scarlet Thread Scripture – *Just as you do not know the path of the wind and how bones are formed in the womb of the pregnant woman, so you do not know the activity of God who makes all things.* **Ecclesiastes 11:5**.

Personal Reflection – What attributes do you have that you got from your Father, God?

_____

Prayer and Meditation - Ask the Holy Spirit to reveal what you need to know about Father God/Yourself.

_____

Personal Deliverance – Expect your desire to be more like God as you seek Him. As He becomes center of your life, others will be removed.

_____

Personal Renewal and Confession - This crossroad can and is removed. There is only one narrow road to Jesus. Baggage keeps us from our destiny. Don't allow it. Recognize just how special you are. Let's free up our souls.

_____

Prayer and Meditation - Ask the Holy Spirit to reveal what you need to know. Let Him lovingly expose the truth. Ask him to help you be more like God.

_____

JOURNAL - Write Your GENETIC STORY

_____

_____

_____

_____

_____

_____

_____

_____

_____

_____

_____

_____

_____

_____

_____

JOURNAL - Write Your GENETIC STORY

_____

_____

_____

_____

_____

_____

_____

_____

_____

_____

_____

_____

_____

_____

_____

_____

_____

Chapter 4

CAPTIVITY ON THE JOURNEY

POST-TRAUMATIC STRESS

It had to have been a very distressing time for my young mother. This was a major tragic life event away from her home, two children, and a husband, my belated, loving father, Henry E. Harris.

My mother lived her early years in a section of Washington that was extremely overpopulated as I mentioned earlier. Several cities in the United States had these outbreaks of Tuberculosis during that time. It is sad that this disease affected my family as it did. We are aware my mother had it, but we don't know for sure if her mother also had T.B. She was severely ill as well.

In this chapter, I will share some of my most devastating medical issues that occurred in my early life and how these issues were signs of future medical problems that would affect my adult life and showed up in many symptoms and illness. I will also share some of the people and treatments and non-tradition-al remedies I was introduced to.

Most of these medical issues were connected to what I experienced at conception. They are genetic and epi-genetic or environmental occurrences. I was held captive in an unseen prison cell without visible bars. The worst part is that I didn't know it or how to get out. As I look back at these events as they began to unfold, God was really showing me a way out. Praise God!

Wherefore he saith,
When he ascended up on high, he led captivity
captive and gave gifts unto men. Ephesians 4:8

I was definitely held captive and I know my mother was. The world has systems in place that can trap us and place us in bondage. We can be captive for many years. It is time to root these issues up and cast them out.

Jesus did it all when He went into the grave and took back the keys to the kingdom. WE ARE FREE!

THE STRESS CONNECTION

The immune system is defined by the National Cancer Institute as a complex system of cells, organs, and tissues that protect the body from bacteria, viruses, and micro-organisms that try to invade it.

> **STRESS**
> c: a physical, chemical, or emotional factor that causes bodily or mental tension and may be a factor in disease causation
> https://www.merriam-webster.com/dictionary/stress

There is a definite connection as demonstrated in my mother's health and mine. I believe I inherited stress from birth. I was, as I mentioned, in her womb for the entire nine months and I knew she feared greatly of the return of Tuberculosis.

I was conceived in December of 1951 and born on September 24, 1952. My family told me that I was a persistently crying infant. So much that I was nick-named "Cry Baby." Why was I crying so much? I asked the Lord because no one else seemed to know why I was crying. God told me "You were in pain."

> **Stress suppresses immune system function and that, over time, the immune system does not adapt but instead continues to wear away.**
>
> *How Does Stress Affect the Immune System? by TRACI JOY Last Updated: Aug 14, 2017 Psychological Bulletin, November 1990*

I was born with a lowered immune system from my mother. She could not pass on to me a strong immune system if she no longer had one. After, years of antibiotics and stress, her system was suppressed or not strong or healthy. She needed antibiotics to kill off bad bugs in her body but, they also killed the good bacteria.

On top of isolation, fears, anxiety, and stress. As a result, I was born with lowered good bacteria in my tiny body and I had to fight for my health and wellbeing.

Science has discovered that prolonged wearing away of the immune system is connected to other problems such as other autoimmune disorders, diabetes, HIV, cancer, etc.

What did my faulty immune system look like as an infant? As I cried constantly, my grandparents held me and walked the floors with me often and for hours at a time, especially at night. I was eventually diagnosed as a colicky baby. Colic was and still is considered severe pain in the intestines that is seen in babies. The cause is unknown. I had to inquire of the Lord for the answer.

I was in pain in my little belly and this started shortly after birth. My immune system was weakened, and I cried for hours at a time in pain. I would have bloating, gas, and pain because I couldn't digest milk well. My mother couldn't breastfeed.

Our immune systems are constantly working to find and destroy foreign invaders just like a little army or better, a big army, all geared up when it is healthy. I call this team of warriors "My Intercessors" within my body.

The body has over 80% fighters that are located in the intestines. Their job is to kill and destroy the enemy pathogens or invaders that come in to take over the body as their own.

After birth, a baby's immune system doesn't fully mature until after eight days or so after birth. Until that time, I was covered and protected by my mother's immune system. As a result of weakened fighters in her body, I adopted my own weakening fighters in my tiny body. I had many things working against me. Besides colic, I also had pain, anxiety, fear, hunger, etc.

Thine eyes did see my substance, yet being unperfect; and in thy book all my members were written, which in continuance were fashioned, when as yet there was none of them.
Psalm 139:16

My little body wasn't even formed yet. God wrote my genetic blueprint in each of my cells, what I would look like from the inside out. In spite of my imperfections, "I am wonderfully and magnificently made." Amazing!

STRESS AND SEPARATION ANXIETY

Another area I like to share is separation anxiety. After my mother was readmitted into the hospital when I was a few months old, I developed anxiety. It is a normal process of growth and development in infants and usually lasts until about two years of age. However, for me, it greatly exceeded that age.

> **Scientists have found that very high levels of stress in the mother can also overwhelm the barrier enzyme in the placenta, allowing the stress hormone cortisol to cross into the fetus's brain.**
>
> THE TELEGRAPH by Richard Gray, Science Correspondent 7:10AM BST 14 Jul 2013

I cried like a baby each morning when it was time to go to school. That 6-month-old baby kept reappearing. My Aunt Shirley would take me to school, she would tell me to stay in my class and stop crying.

As soon as I got to school I cried continually until the principal would make my Aunt Shirley get out of her class and walk me home. This occurred every day in pre-kindergarten until they actually put me out of school. Can you imagine being expelled from school at 4 years old? This happened again in kindergarten.

Again, in the first grade but, by then I was made to stay in school and suffer through it. I was, indeed, a special child. I don't think anyone understood what was wrong with me. I was in pain and still grieving because of the loss of my mother during my first few years of life.

LOW SELF-ESTEEM

I had such difficulty in school and with making friends. As I stated previously, I failed pre-kindergarten and could not adjust to kindergarten or first grade very well. Being in school and away from Grandma was horrible to me. I attended Stevens Elementary School in Northwest Washington, DC. and I remember being punished for crying in class. Actually, I cried all the way to school. I did not feel good about myself.

> **Symptoms of Low Self-Esteem** - Fear & Anxiety are the cornerstones of low self-esteem. Those who suffer from low self-esteem experience extreme fear and anxiety frequently. Believing that there is something innately wrong with themselves, these low self-esteem sufferers experience self-esteem attacks (often called panic attacks) when they do something they deem to have been stupid, something they think others have noticed, and something that confirms their own feelings of inadequacy, incompetence, being undeserving or unlovable.
>
> http://getesteem.com/lse-symptoms/symptom-details.html

When I would cry in class, I remember the teacher and principal would try to get me to settle down. On several occasions, I was taken to the back of the coat closet. I had to hold out my hand to get hit on the hand with the ruler several times to make me behave. I was labeled a behavior problem child, and I just cried more.

No one understood why I was crying they just wanted me to be quiet and sit down like the other children. What was really going on inside of me? Why was I so upset to leave home?

> **Depression:** Low self-esteem is the underlying cause of much of the depression people suffer. They feel that there are things they can't do well, especially as it concerns social skills, being successful, initiating and maintaining relationships, or having the courage to try new things. As a result, they often feel hopeless about their situation and about the future.
> http://getesteem.com/lse-symptoms/symptom-details.html

When I look at myself and what I was going through, I can now see the connection between my fears, anxiety, and depression and how they affected my early life.

As I already mentioned, my problems of fear and anxiety were the foundation as to why I felt so unloved and unwanted.

I remember trying to learn to joke. That didn't work because I had a strange sense of humor. I wanted to curse and say bad words but I sounded out of place. I just didn't know how to fit in.

THE POWER OF WORDS

The words I remembered hearing were, "You are dumb." "You are stupid." "You are a problem." These words kept repeating internally throughout my school-age years. Words are a creative force. We can speak life or death into the lives of others.

Death and life are in the power of the tongue: and they that love it shall eat the fruit thereof.
Proverbs 18:21

When I was in school from the 4th to the 8th grade, I made "F's," "D's," and "C's" in school. I was living the words spoken to and over me. I came in agreement with what others said about me, I called myself "Dumb."

And the tongue is a fire, a world of iniquity: so is the tongue among our members, that it defileth the whole body, and setteth on fire the course of nature; and it is set on fire of hell.
James 3:6

Many of the negative words I received probably came from being teased by others at school because I kept crying. I felt fearful at school. My own self-talk and what others said about me really affected me in a negative way.

I was grown and in college before I even realized I could think more positively about myself. It took the power of God to remove those images embedded in my mind.

TONSILLITIS

I started having infections in my throat when I was about nine years old. I was attending Davis Elementary School at the time in Southeast DC.

My mother was finally well, and my family moved into our own place in subsidized housing in Southeast Washington, D.C. I used to have a sore throat quite often. I also learned to take advantage of the situation and when I didn't want to go to school, I would play like I had a sore throat. That got me a lot of attention from my mother and I enjoyed that.

> At the back of your throat, two masses of tissue called **tonsils** act as filters, trapping germs that could otherwise enter your airways and cause infection. They also produce antibodies to fight infection. But sometimes the **tonsils** themselves become infected. Overwhelmed by bacteria or viruses, they swell and become inflamed, a condition known as **tonsillitis.**
>
> https://www.webmd.com/oral-health/guide/tonsillitis-symptoms-causes-and-treatments#1

Removing tonsils was very popular in the 1960's in America. I was a part of that experience. My immune system was already compromised and removal of my tonsils made me even more susceptible to other diseases. My throat soreness occurred so often that I had to have surgery to remove my tonsils and adenoids. That was quite an experience.

When I woke up, it was all over, and my mother took me home that same day. I had a chance to stay home with my mother, eat ice cream, soup, and drink tea and ginger ale, and be her baby for about two weeks. What a joy!

ALLERGIES

I suffered from allergies pretty badly. I was allergic to dust, pollen, changes in the seasons etc. I also had the worst allergy to crab and shrimp. A shellfish allergy as a small child. Being raised in Washington, DC., you could not go to a house party in those days and not eat crabs. I would get sick almost immediately after breathing the air in the room with the aroma of crabs. My mother would have to put me in a tube of ice cold water and salt to get the whelps and swelling to go down on my skin. After an attack, my eyes remained swollen for about 2 more days.

Allergies and asthma may start in your gut. Upset the gut's natural mix of helpful bacteria and fungi, and allergies and asthma may develop.

According to researchers, the rates of allergies and asthma have increased. They say this correlates with increasing antibiotic use and possibly relates to the hygiene theory. This may mean that modern practices of sanitation could deprive people of defenses needed to prevent asthma and allergies. A Healthy Gut May Resist Allergies, Asthma

Keeping Helpful Bacteria and Fungi in Balance Is Key, Say Researchers

The allergies were resolved about 25 years ago. I was listening to a morning radio show with Kathy Hughes. Her guest was Dick Gregory. The WOL family listeners were doing a seven-day cleanse. I decided to do it too. I had nothing to lose. After all, I was going to an allergist as usual and taking allergy injections in my arms twice a week. In between, I was taking some type of antihistamine every two hours just to breath. Life was some kind of miserable.

I started the cleanse with my first colonic. I went to the local health food store and got my smoothies every other day and that is how I existed for six and a half days until my body said "stop."

It was a life-changing experience and I felt a new-ness in my health for the first time in my life. I woke up the day after the cleanse with renewed energy, glowing from the inside out.

I was so excited, I wanted to become a Wholistic Health Doctor. It was like being on fire for the Gospel and telling everyone I saw about the good news of changing your health and adding years to your life. However, the only person who was excited about cleansing the colon to improved health was ME!

After the cleanse, I tested my body by eating those crabs, shrimp, and lobster I so desired. I never had to get the injection again and I only have to take a very mild antihistamine once or twice a year. Praise God!

DEPRESSION

Sharing mother's stress in the womb leaves children prone to depression. Scientists claim to have unravelled why some people are more prone to suffering from anxiety and depression than others – they shared their mother's stress in the womb.

THE TELEGRAPH by Richard Gray,
Science Correspondent 7:10AM BST 14 Jul 2013

I still cried often, and felt sad and unloved, in spite of the wonderful love from my grandmother and grandfather. My grandfather was Walter Ruffin. He wasn't my natural grandfather but, he really loved me. I remember, he would call me "Little Baby."

The sadness accompanied by low self-esteem continued throughout my young adult life and I just didn't understand why I felt sad so often. I felt worthless and I couldn't even look you in the eyes when I talked to you.

I would always get depressed on my birthday. It was the worst time of the year. I would get very anxious and cry. I did really understand but I believed that it was related to my mother not being there for so many of my birthdays. I also don't remember ever having a birthday party. Last, of all, my sadness could have been related to my actual birth and I didn't like my life very much. I was definitely clinically depressed.

I remember when I was 24 years old, married with two small children, and living in Fayetteville, North Carolina. Yet, I was still crying quite often.

One day my husband said something to me that wasn't too bad, and I cried like a baby. He asked me, "Why do you cry all the time?" Then he walked out of the house. I couldn't answer that question because I didn't really know or paid it much attention.

By that time crying, was a part of my ordinary life. I functioned as a "crying addict" and I didn't know it was depression. In fact, I am just realizing it as I am writing this chapter. There is great power in journaling and shedding the light on those things that got us caught up. It is time to get rid of those weights that we were holding on to for no reason. We all have the ability to cancel all hindrances in our life through Christ Jesus.

Wherefore seeing we also are compassed about with so great a cloud of witnesses, let us lay aside every weight and the sin which doth so easily beset us, and let us run with patience the race that is set before us.
Hebrews 12:1

What exactly are these weights? The Hebrew writer is saying that its anything that is hindering our Christian progress. It the carrying of excess baggage of attitudes, emotions or feeling or fears. It is the sin that we hold on to, whatever we are addicted to, or weakened by.

I was finally ready to start digging deeper into my life and discover what was the true cause of my feelings and insecurities.

My mother had passed away by this time, so I got on the phone to call my Aunt Ruth and Aunt Shirley. I needed to know the reason why I cried so much and why the family called me "Cry Baby." I had questions.

The answer changed my life permanently. Remember, I told you about my pre-birth experience. Well, those fears, anxieties, and grief were still present in my spirit and soul.

For nothing is secret, that shall not be made manifest; neither anything hid, that shall not be known and come abroad.
Luke 8:17

All of this was before I accepted Jesus Christ as My Lord and Savior. I know God was cleaning me up for my future. Once I finished my investigation, I "JUST STOPPED CRYING." That was it!

PRE-ECLAMPSIA

By the time I was a teenager, I had a strong and harmful desire for junk food. I loved chips, cookies, chocolate, and etc. The cravings were overwhelming at times. I would sneak the goodies and I didn't want to eat my dinner. By the way, I still hating those green, leafy, healthy vegetables. I did not connect the cravings with what was going on inside my gut.

Remember, I was born with a lowered immune system. The symptoms were all there from the beginning. I had colic, frequent infections, lots of antibiotics, a poor appetite for healthy foods, a strong desire for junk food, low weight, emotional instability, fears, stress and anxieties, low self-esteem, and depression. All related to a lower immune system.

> **A report in the November 1990 edition of Psychological Bulletin, states that stress suppresses immune system function and that, over time, the immune system does not adapt but instead continues to wear away. What was intended to protect the body, begins to harm it when unregulated. The effect of stress on the immune system has been linked to cancer, AIDS and other autoimmune disorders.**
>
> http://www.livestrong.com/article/22689-stress-affect-immune-system

On top of it all, I became a teenage mother at 17. I knew then I had to change. It was time to learn about food so that my children could be healthier than I was. I did not want them to suffer later in life because of my ignorance. I felt like I needed to save them. From what? I wasn't sure.

I had a difficult pregnancy and was diagnosed with pre-eclampsia. My blood sugar rose during my pregnancy. They didn't allow me to have strong labor pains to prevent my blood pressure from elevating. I had excellent care at D.C. General Hospital at that time.

After the birth of my son, I changed tremendously. I grew up quickly because I had a baby to love and care for. I was a good mother even though I was a teenager. I could finally give love to another person. I held on to him so much. I protected and loved my baby and kept him close to me at all times. I was so proud to be a mother and I didn't want him out of my sight. This was related to my own experience with separating anxiety.

> Preeclampsia is a pregnancy complication character-ized by high blood pressure and signs of damage to another organ system, most often the liver and kidneys. Preeclampsia usually begins after 20 weeks of pregnancy in women whose blood pressure had been normal. Even a slight rise in blood pressure may be a sign of preeclampsia.
>
> http://www.mayoclinic.org/diseases-conditions/preeclampsia/symptoms-causes/syc-20355745

POST-PARTUM DEPRESSION

I had my last child at age 20. My daughter was a beau-tiful baby. I had been a mother now for 3 years and enjoyed motherhood. This time I was married and a homemaker. We were a military family living off base in Fayetteville. My baby girl was born at Womack Army Hospital. That was my life's desire, to have many child-ren and raise them well.

I didn't expect the prolonged labor I had that time since I wasn't allowed to experience it with my first child because of pre-eclampsia. I ate much healthier during the pregnancy and gained the proper amount of weight. I had all the prenatal checks and thought it was going to be a beautiful experience.

Well, first of all, I was in labor for about 48 hours. My husband was in and out of my room. It was hard for him to handle. I remember crying out for drugs to stop the pain. I was finally given an injection of Demerol to help with the pain for about an hour. Once the medication wore off, I was on my own and the pain was tremendous.

Finally, I delivered. I was too exhausted to hold my baby and I didn't want her to stay in the room with me at night. I felt guilty because I couldn't jump back to motherhood. All I wanted to do was sleep. The depression set in. I was so disappointed with the delivery because I had worked so hard to enjoy the pregnancy and have a good delivery. I ate healthier, rested, and was mentally and physically well. However, I felt like an exhausted failure.

My husband helped me when I went home after the two-night stay, but I should have stayed longer in the hospital. My mother had been deceased for about five years at that time. If you ever needed your mother, you certainly need her during childbirth. My depression increased.

Postpartum Depression:
Depression after delivery **affects 1 in 10 mothers**. *Here, symptoms are similar to above, but with greater intensity. Feelings of hopelessness and helplessness are present. One may experience intense exhaustion and sluggishness, confusion, poor concentration, overconcern for the baby or a lack of interest, guilt, feelings of worthlessness, fear of harming the baby or self. These symptoms may appear within days after delivery or may not show up until several months after delivery, and can last for several months unless addressed and treated.*

Depression: A Christian Response Nan Giordano, M.A., L.P.C. Licensed Professional Counselor

I was able to do the basics in my home. I provided for my children, but I wasn't able to give them the full attention they needed. I would hold them but not like I really knew I needed to. I was so disappointed in myself and failing at my greatest goal in life, motherhood.

I could not connect the dots at that time due to my overall emotional health being related to my immune system. When I think about it now, my newborn baby needed me, and I could not give her the proper bonding she desperately needed. Life cycle repeated itself.

Depression for a long period of time is considered clinical depression and should be treated. I wasn't diagnosed or treated, and the depression lasted about a year.

How the Immune System Influences Psychiatric Disorders:

In recent years there has been an increasing awareness of the close connection between physiological states and mental health. New findings suggest the mind-body relationship is even more direct than previously imagined and suggest a potential new target for treatment: the immune system. Until recently, it was believed that the brain is "immune-privileged," operating separately from the peripheral immune system (that of the rest of the body) with minimal interaction between the two.

Tori Rodriguez, MA, LPC
November 03, 2015 http://www.psychiatryadvisor.com/mood-disorders/mental-health-immune-inflammation-depression/article/451482/

I began to resume my normal behaviors. I never really fell that deeply into depression again. I changed my mind about all the babies I once wanted and realized that my spirit, soul, or body wasn't prepared for it.

I could go on and on with my life events, but I wanted you to see the connections that occurred throughout my life. As you can see, I had many roadblocks. These things did distract and delayed me from my purpose and had to be exposed. In the next chapter, I will take these very symptoms to connect to my 50's and how I got the title of *50 Fat and Frustrated.*

Allow God to minister to you concerning the events in your life. Pay attention, even to things that don't seem important because that could be the very thing that can change the path of your life and bring deliverance. Then write your story as God reveals a new journey in Christ Jesus. Be Blessed!

"For nothing is secret, that shall not be made manifest; neither anything hid, that shall not be known and come abroad."
Luke 8:17

ROADMAP TO VICTORY!

<u>Scarlet Thread Scripture</u> – How is the Lord speaking to you in this scripture?

_____

_____

<u>Personal Reflection</u> – Are you aware of any area that held you captive in any way? Do you remember any specific symptoms or medical problems? Emergency visits or incidents or accidents for yourself or your family members or friends. Frequent colds or flu. Anxiety or fears, emotions or pain. Make the phone call or visit. If you are adopted, ask you special parents or look at your birth record if desired. What is the Holy Spirit revealing to you? Is there anything that is in your way that keeps you going in a cycle or stunting your growth in any area of life?

_____

<u>Prayer and Meditation</u> - Ask the Holy Spirit to reveal what you need to know. Let Him lovingly expose the truth.

_____

<u>Personal Deliverance</u> - Once exposed or taken out of darkness, the Lord will remove its power. You will have peace. Receive peace.

_____

<u>Personal Renewal and Confession</u> - This crossroad can and is removed. There is only one narrow road to Jesus. Baggage keeps us from our destiny. Don't allow it. Recognize just how special you are. Let free up your soul.

_____

JOURNAL - Write Your GENETIC STORY

_____

_____

_____

_____

_____

_____

_____

_____

_____

_____

_____

_____

_____

_____

JOURNAL - Write Your GENETIC STORY

_____

_____

_____

_____

_____

_____

_____

_____

_____

_____

_____

_____

_____

_____

_____

_____

Chapter 5

THE SCARLET THREAD

In the book of Joshua, Chapter 6, is the story of how the Scarlet Threads worked for Rahab and represented the blood of the Passover lamb and a symbol of the blood of Christ. The Scarlet Threads also represent God's mercy and forgiveness.

The scarlet thread began in my life before conception and followed me all the days of my life, even before Christ. I will share the scriptures God gives me that demonstrated how the blood of Jesus has always protected me.

I needed some answers on how I even survived from the beginning. The odds were not in my favor but, God knew my situation and had other plans.

Before I formed you in the womb I knew] you, before you were born I set you apart. Jeremiah 1:5 NIV

God knew me when I was just a thought in His mind and before the creation of the world. He set the time for conception and then birthed. God placed everything I needed and who I am to be inside of me. Then assigned my parents.

God understood and knew with intimacy what my pre-life in time would be. This is the place inside my mother's womb where I transitioned to prepare for birth. And yet, He still placed me in the womb of my mother even though her life was compromised.

In the 1950's couples did not exactly plan to have children, they just had them. This was before contraceptives were efficient. The time before birth control pills was established or widely used.

That means God really selected me for that time and season to be born. Many would wonder why God would do that? Why, in an environment that could harm an embryo?

My answer, from the Lord, is the "Scarlet Thread." The blood of Jesus protected me from conception to delivery. This was indication of His love and protection for me. These scriptures are like tiny pieces of a thin red thread that are hardly seen by the naked eye but, God is revealing by His Spirit.

Scarlet Thread Scriptures

As I began to look further at what I call my Natural Inheritance, the Lord began to speak me. Scarlet Thread Scriptures;

**And they saw the God of Israel:
and there was under his feet as it were a paved
work of a sapphire-stone, and as it were the body
of heaven in his clearness.**
Exodus 24:10

Father God presented himself as a sapphire stone. How Awesome! The Lord God is saying to me, **"I am your birthright. You have every right to come** before me. There is a clear vision of who I am to you and you to Me. See Me through the eyes of sapphire high and lifted up. Lift up your head and walk in My Glory." God revealed Himself to me clearly and in love. He wanted me to know how He has always been with me even from the beginning of time.

The Scarlet Scripture Reveals Jesus
Even in Your Darkest Seasons.

GWENDOLYN Listen

to Me, O islands,
And pay attention, you peoples from afar.
The **LORD** called Me from the womb;
From the body of My mother He named Me."
Isaiah 49:1

I believe Father God named me, "Gwendolyn."

A name for girls has its root in Welsh, and the name Gwendolyn means "fair bow; blessed ring".

Associated with **fair (beautiful)**, **blessed**

http://www.thinkbabynames.com/meaning/0/Gwendo ly n#7xXV7aFy76KCTi6Z.99

- I am idealistic, with a great imagination, intuitive, and spiritual.
- I seek and desire spiritual truth in the Word of God, and I depend on hearing from the Holy Spirit.
- I am philosophical or spend time in the study of the fundamental nature of knowledge God's way.
- I spend time devoted to studying the Bible, science, and medicine.

MY BIRTH MONTH

Who hath measured the waters in the hollow of his hand, and meted out heaven with the span, and comprehended the dust of the earth in a measure, and weighed the mountains in scales, and the hills in a balance?
Isaiah 40:12

I was born in the month of September. The birth month is the Libra sign. Libra means balanced. This verse describes how God measured the waters, the heavens, and counted the dust and weighed them. Then, he weighed the mountains and hills.

There are four symbols in Libra; they are;

1. **Libra: the scales;**
2. **Crux: the Southern Cross;**
3. **The Victim; a slain animal, and**
4. **Corona Borealis; a crown.**
   Signs in the Heavens by Marilyn Hickey

SAPPHIRE STONE

And above the firmament that was over their heads was the likeness of a throne as the appearance of a sapphire stone: and upon the likeness of the throne was the likeness as the appearance of a man above upon it.
Ezekiel 1:24, 26

As I looked at the month, date, and time of my birth, I realized there was a connection with the systems God has placed in the Word. The Lord began to reveal to me a few connections that were important to understanding His times and seasons as it is related to when we are born. I believe this is an oversight of many Christians, so I am sharing a few pieces of the pie, so you can see what God revealed to me.

My birthstone is sapphire or lapis lazuli in Ancient Hebrew Name; The Brightened Stone. It is one of the hardest stones next to diamond. This Hebrew name comes from the word *saphar*, to be made beautiful and radiant after removing the outer discoloration by scratching or scraping. Then polished to perfection. Sapphire also means **to inscribe, to write**.

I often wondered why I always had a desire to write. From a young child of about 7 years old, I started writing. I would write stories or read my sister's books and add my version, or, I would listen to old songs my parents used to play and write the words.

For Christmas, I got a record player. My parents cultivated the gift. Praise God!

I also received a prophet word that I would write as the Lord downloaded what He wanted me to write. This prophetic word was about 15 years ago. I am just publishing my first book. There were many stumbling blocks in my path. Now I am in my time and season.

Cultivate Your Children's Gifts. They are Recognized by Desire.

I must confess, initially, when the Lord led me to write about my birthstone I wasn't quite ready to add this to my book, however, God kept downloading information to me.

Father God wanted me to know in scripture; when, where, and how my birthstone and birth timing is connected and the significance of it. Of course, it's all about Jesus and how He is revealing Himself to us. I can see a reflection of myself in the Glory of my Father and His creation. It is related to my purpose and my passion that will ultimately direct me to my destiny.

My birthstone gives me that extra stepping stone to understand more about who I am and who God intended me to be. It is a prophetic sign of my purpose. It is a fresh revelation for me. How wonderful it is to see my prophesied gifts written in the Word of God. Follow the path and allow the Holy Spirit to open your eyes to see your purpose with accuracy. The scripture in Genesis 1 is foundational.

**And God said, Let there be lights in the
firmament of the heaven to divide the day from
the night; and let them be for signs, and for
seasons, and for days, and years.**
Genesis 1:14

In this verse, got a clearer understanding concerning the study of my birthrights. When it comes to my birthstone, birthday, heritage, and birth position, this information was needed. We are living in a time in when we need to understand what God is doing however, and whenever, he chooses to reveal Himself. This is one of the methods He uses.

We should be aware of the increase in interest from the world's point of view on anything by studying and confirming scripture.

Look at what is happening around us in God's creation. Whatever the world is focused on should be a clue that we should pay attention and inquire of the Lord.

God opened my eyes to see that we are missing a lot about what He has done and is doing in His creation. I'm excited about learning more about the heavens and earth, and how God is working throughout to give us the signs so we can understand what He is currently doing and revealing. We also need to know that these things are not just newly made but are already in the plan of God.

For instance, it is already known by science when the constellations will be in a certain arrangement for thousands of years. It wasn't a new prediction that the eclipse was occurring in the United States on August

21, 2017, that went across the United States. The next one is happening in seven years. There is already an appointed time and the season.

He appointed the moon for seasons: the sun knoweth his going down. Thou makest darkness, and it is night: wherein all the beasts of the forest do creep forth.
Psalm 104:19, 20

When I hear about natural occurrences in the earth, it's usually from an astrologist. The job of astrology is to give us a different view of what God is saying. Only God can tell us about what He is actively doing in the Earth realm, and it is confirmed in His creation and proved in His Word.

There is an enemy who is behind the work of astrology. His job is to take credit and pervert the Word of God. That is to misdirect or delay purpose and destiny. He just twists and corrupts the Word of God. Astronomy is seldom, if at all, taught in the church but, it is throughout the Bible. One thing for sure, I was greatly pleased by this spiritual connection.

**He appointed the moon for seasons:
the sun knoweth his going down.**
Psalm 104:19

Astrology

1 archaic: astrology

1. *2*: the divination of the supposed influences of the stars and planets on human affairs and terrestrial events by their positions and aspects

https://www.merriam-webster.com/dictionary/astrology

I have seen many signs and wonders almost daily. I often look for them in the sky. They represent a full spectrum of God's timing and season in the earth.

Why do Christians ignore this reality and insight into the work of His hands?

We give credit to a spirit that is not able to create but a deceiver? We give the credit by not studying the scripture for ourselves concerning unique occurrences often enough.

Even the animal kingdom knows how to live according to the heavens and the moon. Animals use God's direction for habitation. God communicates to mankind and all of His creations through signs and wonders from the heavens.

The Bible gives many examples of how we are supposed to understand and see the beauty of God based on His creation. In fact, these signs are made for us. Animals use and know what's happening around them. Maybe, we need to observe the birds, fish, and deer and notice what God is doing.

I must acknowledge, there is a reason why we might see some truths in the signs from astrology, it's because it the converted truth to get us off course. However, we have the written word to study the reality.

Earthly Signs Reveal God's
Redemption Plan for Mankind in the Earth

Remember, the devil wanted to be like God. There is a vast difference between astrology and astronomy. I will share some of them.

The Mazzeroth

"The band of stars on both sides of this path which is known today as the Zodiac is called the Mazzeroth in Hebrew. The names of these stars, Virgo, Pisces, Capricorn, Leo etc., are familiar to us today, because they are used by astronomers and navigators to designate various areas of the sky. Sadly, they have also been exploited by astrologers for occult purposes which are so very far from the truth. The 12 signs have nothing to say about man, however they do have a great deal to say about God's plan of redemption for mankind - from the virgin birth (Virgo) to the triumph of the Lion of the Tribe of Judah (Leo)!

"Astronomy," *Encyclopedia Judaica*. Jerusalem: Encyclopedia Judaica & New York: Macmillan, 1971-72. 3:795-807.

It is a blessing in knowing our God is speaking to us in many ways including through creation. We should always know what God is doing in the spiritual realm as well as the natural. It is the desire of Jesus to keep us informed. We must stay awake, hear, see, and receive from the Lord.

**Watch ye therefore, and pray always,
that ye may be accounted worthy to escape all
these things that shall come to pass, and to stand
before the Son of man.**
Luke 21:36

What exactly is a sign anyway and how do we recognize them as signs? I see signs in the sky often. I saw angels, and what looked like the face of Jesus years ago. It was probably about 15 years ago. It was a clear vision.

Last fall and winter, almost daily, the sky outside of my bedroom was like fire. It was beautiful scenery. I saw these signs and knew they were of God, but I never really inquired of the Lord what He was saying. All I have to do is ASK!

Lexicon: Strong's H226 - *'owth* **Sign, signal**

1. a distinguishing mark
2. banner
3. remembrance
4. miraculous sign
5. omen
6. warning

token, ensign, standard, miracle,
proof(appearing); a signal (literally or
figuratively), as a flag, beacon, monument, omen,
prodigy, evidence, etc.:—mark, miracle, (en-)
sign, token.

https://www.blueletterbible.org/lang/lexicon/lexicon.cfm?Strongs=H226&t=KJV

LIKE A PARABLE

Biblical astronomy is a powerful resource for those who are called and believe in Jesus Christ. We know according to Genesis that God created the heavens and earth. He gives us signs and wonders to communicate to us his plans and purpose. When I studied this for myself, I was greatly encouraged how Gods purpose shinned a little light to reveal my purpose in Him. For we are truly hidden in Christ.

Biblical Astronomy. *This is not to be confused with astrology, which is the study that assumes and attempts to interpret the influence of the heavenly bodies on human affairs.* **Biblical astronomy recognizes that God created the heavens and they are for signs to us.** *They are also the* **origin of our marking of time.**

http://www.watchmanbiblestudy.com/BibleStudies/BiblicalAstro nomy.html

---

For the invisible things of him from the creation of the world are clearly seen, being understood by the things that are made,
Romans 1:20a

God is not creating anymore; He depends on man to do His work on the earth. However, there are many signs, wonders, and miracles that God is still manifesting around us. He is actively communicating to us daily; however, this was set in place at creation. It's like a type of nonverbal or sign language. I think it's time for more serious watching. God established the times and seasons, days and years prophetic signs.

GOD'S ORDER OF TWELVE

God established the world and everything in heaven and earth in divine order. I was excited to learn of my spiritual heritage and I will share some of it with you. God is a God of order. Science can identify the order of times and seasons by the constellation. So should we.

NATURAL HERITAGE

The Lord began to show me my true heritage from the standpoint of my birthright. I found this to be an eye-opener to purpose and destiny. It helped me to understand who I am and my gift.

As I continued to research and study my natural birthright, I tapped into another touch of Glory. The Shekinah Glory of God on my back porch as I was researching and writing about this subject. His presence was life-changing, and this visitation occurred on my back porch on a pleasant Saturday afternoon while writing this chapter.

The presence of God showed up mightily while I was studying for this part of the book. I don't ever remember studying anything with such Anointing and Power of God. I knew I was on the right path. The Lord began to purify me for His presence. I received a divine download of revelation.

Before I realized it, I stepped into another realm of Glory. I had entered the throne room of God. A place where I have visited and have accessed but not quite as often as I should. However, this time, it was a place or a realm I had never been before. This time I entered with a different purpose or assignment from the Lord. I knew God wanted me to be in my place of authority with a fresh anointing and position.

**Expect Immediate Presence
When You Enter Your Natural Inheritance.
God Will Meet You There.**

SCARLET THRED SCRIPTURES

As I began to look further at what I call my Natural Inheritance, the Lord began to reveal and speak to me. These are the Scarlet Thread Scriptures for me.

And they saw the God of Israel: and there was under his feet as it were a paved work of a sapphire-stone, and as it were the body of heaven in his clearness.
Exodus 24:10

Father God presented himself as a sapphire stone. How Awesome! The Lord God is saying to me,

"I am your birthright. You have every right to come before me. There is a clear vision of who I am to you and you to me. See me through the eyes

of sapphire high and lifted up. Lift up your head and walk in my Glory."

God revealed my birthright. I am to know God and have a close relationship with Him. My birthstone sapphire represents how I see Him in His Glory.

ISSACHAR CONNECTION

I discovered my connection to the line of Issachar. My birthstone is sapphire, and it is the color blue. Issachar was from one of the Tribes of Israel. His jewel stone was also sapphire.

My birthstone in Hebrew means, the Brightened Stone. This stone is one of the hardest stones next to the diamond.

I started to think about what I experienced in my younger life. Some of the things I remembered assisted in my fragile image of myself. I was insecure, easy to offend, a timid person with low self-esteem. I remembered that I went through a long process of emotional stabilizing years ago. I see why the process was necessary. I had to change.

Issachar's [stone was] sappir, *and the color of his flag was dark blue [lit. black like kohl], and a sun and a moon were drawn on it, as it is written.*

http://christianhospitality.org/resources/breastplate/birthstones.html

Once I got connected with the Holy Spirit, I began seeing and understand more of my purpose through the eyes of Jesus.

**And of the children of Issachar,
which were men that had understanding of the
times, to know what Israel ought to do; the heads
of them were two hundred, and all their brethren
were at their commandment.**
1 Chronicles 12:33

The sons of Issachar were men of discernment. They had an understanding of the times, and seasons to know what Israel ought to do. It was a large tribe. They were known for their intelligence. Issachar's tribe was a leader among the other tribes. All the brothers listened and followed them. They were men of experience, who knew what needed to be done at all times.

THE BIRTH COLOR BLUE

Blue has been my favorite color since I can remember, especially the medium blue color. Now I have an understanding that blue is a royal color that represents God's Presence.

**And they saw the God of Israel. Under his feet
was something like a pavement made of lapis
lazuli, as bright blue as the sky.**
Exodus 24:10

ROADMAP TO VICTORY!

<u>Scarlet Thread Scripture</u> – What scripture describes your birthright, birthstone, and birth sign?

_____

<u>Personal Reflection</u> – What gifts or abilities do you have in common with your birth description from your birthright?

_____

<u>Prayer and Meditation</u> – Ask God to reveal to you your birthright authority and identity connected to your birthright.

_____

<u>Personal Deliverance</u> – Expect to see yourself like God sees you in complete authority. You will receive encouragement. As He becomes the center of your life, others will be removed.

_____

<u>Personal Renewal and Confession</u> – You now have a greater insight into your calling and plan of God for you in the earth. The stumbling block has been removed permanently. Walk in freedom!

_____

<u>Prayer and Meditation</u> – Agree with the gifts, callings, purpose, and destiny that the Lord revealed concerning you. Take authority.

_____

_____

JOURNAL – Write Your "NATURAL HERITAGE AND SCRIPTURE"

_____

_____

_____

_____

_____

_____

_____

_____

_____

_____

_____

_____

_____

_____

JOURNAL - Write Your "NATURAL HERITAGE AND SCRIPTURE"

_____

_____

_____

_____

_____

_____

_____

_____

_____

_____

_____

_____

_____

_____

_____

_____

_____

Chapter 6

THE MANIFESTATION

It's interesting that when God gave me the title of my book, *50 Fat and Frustrated*, I didn't know where he was going to take me with it. I thought it was just a health informational book, however, it is whole body health. It's total personal health, not just physical.

I will talk about each of these areas I experienced as an infant and how they progressed into my adult life. I will also show you how these conditions presented differently in my life by the time I was between 45 to 50. Life was pretty miserable.

What I was most frustrated about was the aging process and I hadn't completed my assignment. I was very busy at that time working in ministry and my local church and community, however, it was getting harder to maintain. I needed a makeover and only the Lord could do it for me.

I will not only discuss some of my symptoms but some of the solutions that worked for me. Everybody is different, so I am really talking about me. I usually resolved many issues with nontraditional therapies. These therapies worked better than traditional medical treatments for me.

Disclaimer: *None of this information is intended to treat or cure any diseases or medical problems. I am not a medical doctor. This is my autobiography or my story. Everyone is different.*

This information is just to show you what helped me and is for informational purposes only.

MY TEMPLE HEALTH (BODY)

Surely he hath borne our griefs, and carried our sorrows: yet we did esteem him stricken, smitten of God, and afflicted. But he was wounded for our transgressions, he was bruised for our iniquities: the chastisement of our peace was upon him, and with his stripes, we are healed.
Isaiah 53:4-5

I discussed quite a lot about my immune system from birth. These are my gut warriors that help fight off infection and maintain balance and a healthy internal environment. Most of these fighters are located within the intestines.

I inherited a weakened intestinal environment and I didn't like the healthy foods, as a child or teen, therefore, I made my health even worse as I got older. Now we will look at some of the issues and how they progressed as they became chronic or long term.

As I stated, I was a colicky baby and that meant that I had problems in my gut right after birth. As we now know, this could possibly indicate that I had problems digesting food or the formula wasn't digesting so that I could be satisfied. You know how important it is for a baby to get their belly full in order to sleep.

As an adult, I had periods of diverticulitis in my large bowel that cause pain and discomfort. On occasions, these pockets got infected and became extremely painful until I needed treatment. I would fluctuate from diarrhea to constipation at any time. The treatment was usually a low-fiber diet and medication. This problem increased in my mid-forties.

Another gut problem I experienced was irritable bowel syndrome or IBS. This term is very common, and it is related also to abdominal pain and diarrhea.

Yet another issue was extreme Gastroesophageal Reflux Disorder. This term is quite common now days also. Many people have it. It is known as GERD. This condition is also a digestive disorder. I remember it being so bad when I was about 48 that I was hospital-ized for 24 hours to make sure I wasn't having a heart attack. The pain was severed in the middle of my chest. I was put on medication for a year.

I gained 60 pounds by the time I was 50 years old. I had belly fat, fatigue, brain fog, and a lot of forget-fulness. I also started perimenopause symptoms, high cholesterol, and my blood sugar level was out of con-trol. I was truly a mess.

What concerned me most was the belly fat, bloat-ing and diarrhea and/or constipation. I was miserable and frustrated. As you can see, I continued from in-fancy with bowel problems as it related to my immune system throughout my life. The connection was there from the beginning.

MY NATURAL REMEDIES

Since colic is related to the lowered immune system, strengthening the immune system with breast milk, if possible, and/or making your own fermented baby food will help as the child gets older.

My grandmother would make apple butter and other types of fermented food. These foods are probiotics and helped without me even knowing it back then.

I would take probiotics from time to time and it would make me feel better and give me energy. I also started getting very healthy with fewer colds and flu. Prebiotics were a real problem when I was much younger and when I started having my own children I included those healthy, fresh, raw vegetables in our meals. Prebiotics are raw, high fiber food sources that feed the probiotics. I would eat raw, dandelion greens, leeks, lots of onions in my meals, garlic, lots of kale and much more. I would also put them in my smoothies.

I finally got rid of the diverticulitis with a colon cleanse. I would do a cleanse at least twice a year for several years.

Another problem I frequently had was yeast infections. This is extremely common for women and I thought the answer was frequent vaginal cleanses, when, in fact, the douche increased the yeast infections. When I stopped the cleanses, the infections stopped. Yeast infections were another sign that the good bacteria in my body was weakened.

I did a colon cleanse for four days with fasting. I used special herbs and a colonic. The result was successful. I expelled crud, waste, and worms that apparently were inside for a long time. After the cleanse, I increased whole healthy foods and supplements.

I got rid of the reflux in three days with apple cider vinegar and kale smoothies. I learned this magnificent treatment from one of my chiropractor mentors and teachers.

Finally, I maintained my colon health with apple cider vinegar and baking soda. This is an excellent way I cleanse by bowel when needed. Cultured food and drinks like kefir and sauerkraut help. I love to make kombucha fermented drinks.

As a result of years of practice on myself and suggestions and treatments from other practitioners, I am able to maintain my gastrointestinal health well. I lost the 60 pounds, my thoughts cleared up. I gained energy and my blood sugars were controlled depending on what I ate or my activity.

RAM IN THE BUSH/ GRANDMA MAHALA

First of all, I had periods of healing. When I look back, I can clearly see how God was with me. He had people assigned to me to be there and make sure I didn't fall.

My grandmother was a wonderful substitute for me from birth. I would have died as an infant if it hadn't been for her. I just wanted to mention her because she did a wonderful job and I watched her every move.

Mahala Harris was a beautiful and strong woman. I attached to her because she gave me so much attention and love. All I wanted to do was to stay at home with her.

I had such a close relationship with my grandmother and I thought she was my mother. In fact, I called her "Mama" until I was about eight years old and we moved away. I had a wonderful time with grandma. I remember it was just the two of us all day together, all day having fun.

Grandma and I would drink hot tea with cream as we sat in front of the big living room window in our rocking chairs. We would sew quilts by hand and I watched her as she talked to friends or neighbors in the midday.

During those special times together with my grand-mother, I don't remember many sick visits to the hospital for general treatments. Grandmother used the backyard as her pharmacy. She would make her own remedies from plants she grew in her garden. This was my introduction to nontraditional therapies. She made homemade remedies for almost anything—cough syrup from onions, chest rubs from garlic and herbs. Most of all, she fermented beer, wine, apple butter, jelly and jam. I learned a lot from Grandma. These treasures are missing from many cultures today.

Being with grandma not only gave me wisdom and exposed me to many talents and natural treatments, she also provided spiritual and emotional wellbeing.

Now, I am known by my grandchildren as the grandmother that can fix it! They trust that I have the answer to their belly ache, rashes, scrapes, and pains. To God be the glory!

SPIRIT HEALTH

What? know ye not that your body is the temple of the Holy Ghost which is in you, which ye have of God, and ye are not your own? For ye are bought with a price: therefore glorify God in your body, and in your spirit, which are God's.
1 Corinthians 6:19-20

Another area I like to share is separation anxiety. When I was a few months old, I developed anxiety. It is a normal process of growth and development in infants and usually lasts until about two years of age. However, for me, it greatly exceeded that age.

In fact, I always had a nervous stomach. I don't remember when I didn't. While I was doing research for my book, I found out that separation anxiety can affect adults also. I never realized I still had the problem until I started looking at the symptoms. They resemble the symptoms in small children. Researchers now have evidence that adults can suffer with it too. Amazing.

It seems, anxiety has always been an issue with me. A rash on my neck would come and go for years and I just felt anxious almost all the time. I knew whenever I got scared about something, the rash would appear a few days later. I never understood this issue. I remember always feeling anxiety deep inside.

I learned and practiced how to worship God while attending Jericho Baptist Bible School when I was about 50 years old. I'm not talking about clapping my hands and dancing before the Lord. I'm talking about true worship in Spirit and Truth. That's when I experienced for REAL the healing powers of God through worship.

Jesus saith unto her, Woman, believe me, the hour cometh when ye shall neither in this mountain nor yet at Jerusalem, worship the Father. Ye worship ye know not what: we know what we worship: for salvation is of the Jews. But the hour cometh, and now is, when the true worshippers shall worship the Father in spirit and in truth: for the Father seemed such to worship him. God is a Spirit: and they that worship him must worship him in spirit and in truth. The woman saith unto him, I know that the Messiah cometh, which is called Christ: when he is come, he will tell us all things. Jesus saith unto her, I that speak unto thee am he.
John 4:21-26

This scripture explains healing like no other to me. My life has been totally transformed through worship.

Let me share with you the principle of worship as stated above. This kind of worship can't be done in a building, a church, or at a conference. We don't know the saving power of worship God's way until we tap into worship in the spirit and in the truth of who Jesus is and the saving power of deliverance.

The verse also tells us the Father is looking for us to come to Him in this way for our healing and He is the Healer, Hallelujah!

When I became a worshiper, my spirit, soul, and body health turned around. I knew the principle of healing God's way and I would go to the throne for the continued flow of the blood of Jesus. The blood that heals, delivers, and set us free. I am a true worshiper!

Depression was apparent to me. I knew I was depressed at times. It never got as serious as it was after pregnancy, but that spirit would come upon me during crisis events.

How did I get rid of these spiritual issues? My only answer is the Lord. Father God revealed them to me and then took them away. I remember when He was teaching me about depression. The Lord showed me I was coming out of a dark tunnel as I turned my head to look back, I saw a deep dark cave, and I was now on the other side. I had been there for months and didn't realize it.

Another time, I saw what looked like a blanket falling down over my head and before I let it cover me, I rebuked it and it went away. Glory be to God!

**He healeth the broken in heart,
and bindeth up their wounds.**
John 4:3

ANOTHER MOTHER / ABNA REID HALL

I called her "Nana." She picked up raising me right after my mother went home to be with the Lord. God placed her in my life to teach me how to survive and how to be a woman. She was the mother that didn't birth me into the world but thought she did.

Abna Reid Hall stood 5-feet tall in high heels. She was radiantly beautiful, intelligent, spicy, and the most elegant, Christian woman you would ever meet. She lived across the street from us and loved me just as her own. Eventually, she became the grandmother of my children.

We had a unique mother-daughter relationship. I spent a lot of time in her presence as she taught me many important life skills. She took over teaching me how to be a woman. She also taught me to dress, wear makeup, fix my hair, cook, keep a bank account, clean, carry myself as a lady and most of all not to think too highly of myself or "smell myself."

I remember simply watching her every move. She not only taught me natural things but, she prayed me into salvation. I accepted Christ in 1980 at True Vine Missionary Baptist Church in Lompoc, California. I still miss my Nana today.

SOUL HEALTH
MIND-WILL-INTELLECT-EMOTIONS

**"Sticks and stones will break my bones,
but words will never harm me."**

A response to an insult, implying that "You might be hurt able to hurt me by physical force but not by insults."

Origin: 'Sticks and stones may break my bones, but names will never hurt me' is a stock response to verbal bullying in school playgrounds throughout the English-speaking world. It sounds a little antiquated these days and has no doubt been superseded by more streetwise comebacks.

The earliest citation of it that I can find is from an American periodical with a largely black audience, The Christian Recorder, March 1862

Remember the old adage, 'Sticks and stones will break my bones, but words will never harm me'. True courage consists in doing what is right, despite the jeers and sneers of our companions.

The Phrase Finder;
https://www.phrases.org.uk/meanings/sticks-and-stones-may-break-my-bones.html

I internalized the words "dumb," "stupid," "a problem," that I had heard over and over throughout my school-age years. Words are a creative force. Words can make or break you. Well, they certainly broke my will. I was crushed!

Those negative images were embedded in the walls of my soul for years. My self-talk came in agreement with what I heard. I knew I wasn't much and this belief was deep within me.

I had difficulty making friends when I first started school. As I stated previously, I failed pre-kindergarten and could not adjust to kindergarten or first grade very well. I also failed the fourth grade because I was sick often with infections from Tonsillitis. Being in elementary school was not easy for me.

Fear and anxiety was my foundation of low self-esteem. Those who suffer from low self-esteem experience extreme fear and anxiety frequently. I knew that there was really something wrong with me. I was told that I was always doing something stupid. That made me feel more and more inadequate, incompetent, being undeserving or unlovable.

My self-image caused the low self-esteem and my self-talk empowered it. I felt so unworthy even as an adult, I had difficulty looking into your eyes while talking with you. I felt like that little 5-year-old over and over again. I wanted to cry and get away to be alone, but I had to face life and live in society.

In fact, I took a class to learn how to speak in public when I was in nursing school to get over the problem. That's when I learned what was going on within me. I always knew the answers to my problems was in a book, so I started learning. In fact, for the next 20 years.

I finally got rid of the low self-esteem when I got saved. When I learned about what Jesus did for me on the cross, it was over!

Being confident of this very thing, that he, who hath begun a good work in you, will perfect it unto the day of Christ Jesus.
Philippians 1:6

THE TONGUE OF EDUCATORS /
MR. ELLIOTT SMITH

Death and life are in the power of the tongue: and they that love it shall eat the fruit thereof.
Proverbs 18:21

The other person God sent into my life for a short season was my English teacher, Mr. Elliott. He was a teacher at Sousa Junior High School in Southeast Washington.

When I returned to school after my mother passed away, we had an English test. I was just sitting in my seat crying silently. He walked over to me and placed his hands on my shoulder. As I looked up at him he said to me, "I bet you can make a "B" on this test." I said to him, "I can?" He commented, "Yes you can."

And the tongue is a fire, a world of iniquity: so is the tongue among our members, that it defileth the whole body, and setteth on fire the course of nature; and it is set on fire of hell.
James 3:6

It was absolutely amazing what he dared say to me. How could he see a jewel inside of an old deteriorating wooden box? I was shattered and felt defeated in life at 15 because of my "just life" experiences. I'm not blaming anyone, things just happened.

This was my PRE-CHIRST times and season in my life. I didn't even know why I was still alive or on earth.

My life was shattered all over again because my mother passed away! What was going on in my mind?

And he brought me to the door of the court; and when I looked, behold a hole in the wall. Then said he unto me, Son of man, dig now in the wall: and when I had digged in the wall, behold a door.
Ezekiel 8:7-8

I ministered at a women's conference in my church a few years ago on emotional abuse and the Lord showed me how the memory of words embedded in our subconscious soul will bury itself until God reveals and removes it.

Before we are saved, the experiences we have, good and bad are deep inside of us and come back to haunt us. The bad memories will flare up at anything because they have a place of habitation inside of us. The verse above is about sin that was going on and God gave Ezekiel the revelation of the subconscious mind.

This area in the mind is described here as a hole in a wall and Ezekiel was instructed to dig deeper into the wall and what was discovered was another door that leads to another wall.

When words are spoken to us they actually penetrate and are like fire burning deep into the chambers of our mind. Changing the course of our life from the direction of God to destruction. But God has put eternity in our heart or soul when he breathed into us the breath of life and we became a living being.

This eternity is God because our God is Eternal. Therefore, this is the last genetic code I will speak on. We are not an afterthought but, planned and pre-planned from the foundation of the world. We are wired for VICTORY!

NO MORE EXCUSES

What do workers gain from their toil? I have seen the burden God has laid on the human race. He has made everything beautiful in its time. He has also set eternity in the human heart, yet no one can fathom what God has done from beginning to end. I know that there is nothing better for people than to be happy and to do good while they live. That each of them may eat and drink, and find satisfaction in all their toil—this is the gift of God. I know that everything God does will endure forever; nothing can be added to it and nothing taken from it. God does it so that people will fear him.
Ecclesiastes 3:9-14

In conclusion, we see the genetics of God explained clearly. Everything was laid out for mankind before we came into this sinful world, the evil trickery that was done, and the purpose of it.

Most importantly, we see that the Lord Jesus has never left us or forsaken us, as He stated in the Word. We also were able to understand the Scarlet Thread Scriptures that identified Jesus's covering by His blood that continued to flow even in our lost state and wilderness seasons.

When it looked like the enemy had control over my life, in reality, was just a fake stage. You see, I already WON!

God hand-selected our parents to birth us into the world. They had to learn and experience life along the way, they made some mistakes and so did we.

The enemy used our lives to try to kill, steal, and destroy us from our purpose in God by epigenetics or by blocking our heritage in the Lord.

The Lord has a blueprint already established in our genetic makeup. It is already written in our cells. Legal documents or contracts were drafted by our Judge Jesus and established before we were placed into time. It is our covenant and is in our book of purpose and we discover it as God reveals it to each of us.

Therefore, we are counseled one on one and His Word is hidden within our hearts. Just like our purpose is personal and only the Father can reveal it from the inside out.

This purpose is not ours to make up but to discover as we work out our own salvation. God gives us the ministry gifts to assist in the direction of life to help grow us up in the Word. Ultimately, we must develop our intimate relationship with the Father. He will take out the old scripts in our mind and replace them with our destiny in Christ. One-on-one with God is how He will lead and direct us every step of the way to His purpose and Glory.

Finally, I discussed our **Natural Heritage.** The Lord began to show me my true heritage from the standpoint of my birthright. I found this to be an eye-opener to purpose and destiny. It helped me to understand who I am and my gift and how everything was laid before me and I just have to receive and walk in it as I placed Jesus in the center of my life.

It was very encouraging to see Jesus in another way revealing Himself to me. He shined the light into my heart and reflected God in me. Praise the Lord!

**To console those who mourn in Zion,
To give them beauty for ashes, The
oil of joy for mourning,
The garment of praise for the spirit of heaviness;
That they may be called trees of righteousness,
The planting of the LORD,
that He may be glorified."**
Isaiah 61:3 (NKJV)

God summed it up this way: **"The evil works that were sent to stop your destiny in me cannot unless you allow it. I have already given my people every-thing 'pertaining to life and godliness' according to My Word and My Will. Choose life and you will live abundantly in Me and I in you. Without Me, you can do absolutely nothing. Everything made is beauti-fied in its time and season and no man knows the time or season unless I reveal it to him. Eternity that is in your heart is Me and bigger than you can imagine. I have to reveal it to you slowly and surely. My time is not your time and everything you went through is and will be beautiful in its season. I will reveal to you the beauty inside and you will share the**

beauty with others to encourage them so they truly know that I am GOD. I want My people to know and trust Me." Thus, said the Lord God.

How did my teacher, Mr. Elliott, know to speak to me to encourage me? Could God have used him? Was this an example of the "Scarlet Thread." Was this an assignment from God that was intended to clear the roadblocks that were redirecting my life and kept in the wilderness.

I know that many roadblocks were removed and I began to see the manifestations gradually over the years. This began my entrance into the next level of my life.

Mr. Elliott had the audacity to break up the "fallow ground" in my subconscious mind and planted new seeds. He did it in the classroom of an 8th grade middle school.

I was amazed he said that because I never made a "B" in my whole time in school, and only a few "C's." I always thought I had a learning disability, in fact, I know I do. Hopefully, it is unnoticed by now.

God turned that around too. I couldn't imagine this teacher speaking into my life this way. He said some-thing good about me that impacted my world. His words changed my life forever. I made my very first "B" and have been making "A's" and "B's" ever since.

Because of the encouragement of Mr. Elliott, I went on to nursing school. I felt smart, wise, intelligent, and I had a lot to say after that! In fact, I had a goal to get my Ph.D. in Theology, the study of my Maker,

GOD. My average grades in school were "A's" and "B's." To God be all the glory!

**For what may be known about God
is plain to them, because God has made it
plain to them. For since the creation of the world
God's invisible qualities, His eternal power, and
divine nature, have been clearly seen, being
understood from His workmanship, so that men
are without excuse.**
Romans 1:18-19

*IF YOU HAVE NOT MADE THE DECISION TO MAKE
JESUS YOUR LORD AND SAVIOR. NOW IS THE TIME.
ASK HIM NOW TO COME INTO YOUR LIFE AND SAVE
YOU FROM THIS SIN-SICK WORLD, AND HE WILL
TURN YOUR LIFE AROUND!*

Before

After

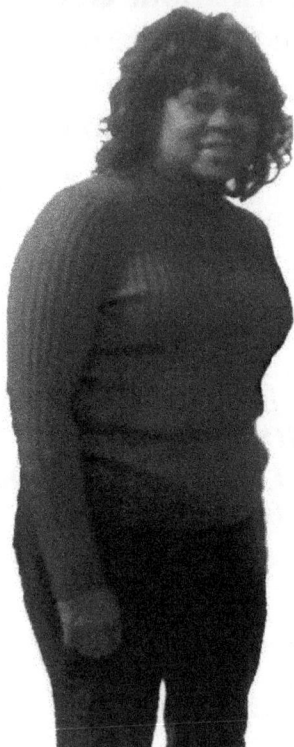
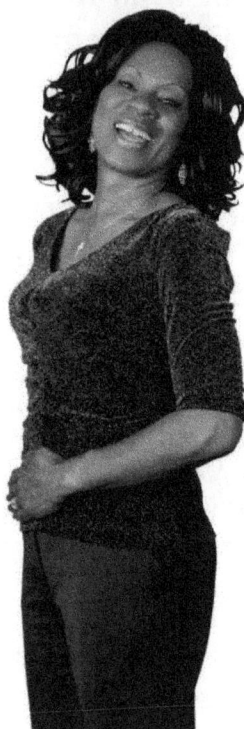

www.ingramcontent.com/pod-product-compliance
Lightning Source LLC
Chambersburg PA
CBHW030023290326
41934CB00005B/464